SELF HEALING GUIDE

I0132325

The accompanying video can be watched at:

http://youtu.be/358XNqIVPoc

Author: Dimitrios Mangioros

Translators: Irene Angelidou, Iole Mangiorou

Production Supervisor: Platon Malliagkas, mediterrabooks.com

© 2015, Dimitrios P. Mangioros

e-mail: acumag@hotmail.com

ISBN 978-960-93-6913-8

Dimitrios P. Mangioros

Neurosurgeon-Acupuncturist

SELF HEALING GUIDE
Learn Self Acupuncture

in combination with

Herbs, Relaxation, Diet, Hydrotherapy

Dedicated

to my family

and

to people who use their knowledge ethically

TABLE OF CONTENTS

Prologue

The purpose of this book is to help even a single person in overcoming an illness, alleviating its symptoms or preventing any such occurrence and maintaining a healthy mind and body.

"The word help is very significant", a professor in the Aristotle University of Thessaloniki used to tell us. "You will be successful medical doctors if you help even a single patient." Prescribing medication, such as a painkiller (aspirin or even something more potent, such as morphine) is significant and helpful, but our fellow people are truly helped when medical doctors devote time to help them realize the real causes of their illness and offer them justified medical treatment with the fewest side effects.

An illness is usually a result of one's lifestyle caused by anxiety, unhealthy diet, lack of physical exercise or bad habits (smoking, alcohol consumption, overmedication, sexual extravagance, lack of sleep, excessive screen time). Sometimes "The sins of the fathers..." are "...visited upon the heads of their children".

We need bright examples that will teach us love, simplicity and the desire for self-improvement. There is not enough space in a book to teach all of the above but I will attempt to convey to you the truth that I have discovered after 25 years of practicing alternative forms of medicine.

For the first time on a global level, it is stated in my book that the Primary Meridians (the main energy routes in the human body) consist of ten vibrating fibers, and the space between them fluctuates in proportion to the yin and yang energy.

For the first time on a global level, the waveform of the energy which is absorbed or emitted from the head of the needle at stimulation or dispersion during acupuncture is analyzed in my book.

For the first time, the Hellenic herbal needles are mentioned and details are provided for their use; I strongly suggest that they should be exported abroad.

For the first time a great number of herbs are classified according to the Empedoclean-Hippocratic doctrine.

After online research, I realized that a book written in English with the words "learn self acupuncture" in the title doesn't exist.

By reading this book carefully, you will see a dramatic decrease in your medical expenses. Visits to your physician will not stop altogether, but they will be fewer; you will take less medication (either because you will not need it or because it will be supplemented with needles) and the periods of absence from work will be reduced dramatically.

You should always remember that your illness must be diagnosed by a medical doctor with the assistance of laboratory and imaging tests, especially if the condition is not easily treatable.

In this book, there is barely any mention of traditional Chinese theory based diagnosis, due to its high complexity. I am no expert and most importantly, I don't want you getting side-tracked by following wrong healing ways.

This book is addressed to everyday people who are looking for help, when they are shipwrecked in the sea of illness. It isn't an encyclopedia of self healing ways. On the contrary, it mentions a few simple, but helpful, things that can be used by all readers.

If you have any question for the proper placing of the needles, a visit to my private medical office, or to a willing, nearby acupuncturist, will help.

This treatise aims to be your friendly guide, a small stepping stone towards changing your way of life and priorities, and it provides you with simple ways of combating anxiety, instructions for a diet as healthy as possible, incentives for physical exercise and for limiting or removing bad habits and finally, instructions on how to take advantage of the natural resources (thermal baths, herbs, herbal needles) God has offered you.

Don't be afraid, try to rely on your strength, dedicate some time and space to self healing and self acupuncture, and never forget that you have been created in the image and likeness of God, which means you have endless potential of spiritual evolution and self healing. You should put your faith in simple therapeutic means, and only when you have exhausted all of them should you proceed to expensive and complex treatments or surgery, which could possibly have serious side-effects.

What is simpler than placing a needle on the spot where you feel pain? If you are afraid or if your child is afraid, stick an adhesive magnet on the particular spot or massage it gently for ten minutes.

I advise you to read the whole book and not just a few pages, because you might make an error in the application of the treatments.

SECTION 1: RELAXATION

Prayer

Prayer is the highest form of spiritual and physical uplifting. With prayer, humans commune their Maker, their roots, and not only do they gain strength, but also inner peace and energy; by expelling negative feelings and thoughts, they are reborn.

Contact with God and his dictates (you shall love your God and you shall love your fellow man as you love yourself), namely with love [the Hellenic word for love is "agape" which derives from the words ago+pan (guide+everything)], "guides" humans everywhere; to become one with nature, one with the universe, and offers them the most effective medicine.

In order to reach deification, to come into direct contact with God, you have to be in tune with His energy, which ascetics achieve through a simple way of life, praying and physical-spiritual fast.

Prayer's most important element is your love towards the Lord. Your mind and body must crave Him.

The right prayer requires as a prerequisite the knowledge of your insignificance and the fact that you converse with the Creator of All Things. Therefore, when praying, you have to be completely focused, in a quiet environment, and with your mind concentrated on the Creator.

It isn't proper to watch TV for hours and then pray right away. Some kind of preparation is needed, like reading a Christian-themed book, taking a hot bath, or having some chamomile tea (matricaria chamomilla).

It is said that the most suitable hour for praying is during the morning service, which in the monasteries of the Holy Mount of Athos starts at 3.30 am.

The insiders speak of an inner, silent, continuous and constant prayer by usually repeating the phrase "show mercy to me, Lord Jesus". You should repeat the same phrase, even if you are praying for other people, because the "me" represents human unity; everyone's Father is the only God, so the problem of your brother is your problem too.

You can begin at night-time, when you have switched off the lights and you are ready to fall asleep, by slowly repeating the phrase "Help me, oh Lord", and by projecting every word as an image in your mind. If other thoughts come to you, you shouldn't drive them away, but, once more, you should concentrate on every word of the prayer.

Your mind must become calmer and, first and foremost, be filled with love and humility, in order to give your body the opportunity to really heal itself. You have to realize that your disposition, thoughts and emotions have a direct effect on it.

When your thoughts are simple, benevolent, positive, optimistic (if a thorn gets in your hand, be glad it didn't get in your eye), compassionate and filled with faith towards God, then not only will you have a catalytic effect on the illness, but, as the gospel proclaims, you can also have such a great effect on your environment, that you might even move mountains.

When you are tormented by thoughts, guilt, anxiety and fear, you should change courses and visit your spiritual mentor. You have to pick them only after a careful search, and, when they speak, they have to radiate Christian love. Most of the time, you are in need of penance (with an aching heart, a confession on the lips, and on the way to correcting your life) and prayer.

It's the spirit that first falls ill, then your energy, and subsequently, the body. Because of this, you have to pray, first and foremost. You may ask God what you wish, but you have to respect His previous dictates, and allow the lift of prayer to take you not where you want to go, but where you ought to be. This relationship goes two ways, despite His boundless love towards all of His children.

Illness doesn't exist as God's punishment, but as a means of change; to limit selfishness, to raise awareness of humanity's fragile nature and teach the virtue of patience, which strengthens faith towards God.

Many times, illness is the road towards a great adventure, through which you could discover the true meaning of life. You realize the futility of coveting material goods or offices, but also the worth of a walk, a simple food prepared with love, a song, friendship, a good deed. There is no joy without pain, and there is no victory without war. A lot of blood is split in war; Jesus Christ is the master craftsman who fought the Devil and utterly defeated him.

In the Holy Mount of Athos, they say that illness is a visit from God.

At times, an illness aims at the spiritual betterment of relatives or friends. Other times, an illness aims to expose environmental pollution. At times, "the sins of the fathers are visited upon the children"; there might be recurring congenital or genetic disorders due to problems that first appeared up to 7 generations ago.

When Jesus' disciples asked him if a man who had been born blind was being punished for his parents' sins, the Lord answered: "Neither had this man sinned, nor his parents; but it was so that the works of God might be displayed in him."

An illness can be beneficial only if you praise and thank God during its course. Humans have been given the power to heal psychic pain through physical ordeal.

A person grows up with the ambition to gain a respectable position in society, and material goods, equating both with happiness. It's important to avoid creating artificial consumeristic needs, be frugal, and value simplicity in your life and character. When you forget your life's purpose and become greedy, then you become anxious to gain more and maintain them.

The pursuit of material goods and social recognition causes anxiety and this is how the vicious circle of mental and physical illness begins. Anxiety leads to physical exhaustion and drains your energy, things which heighten anxiety, because subconsciously you realize that your diminishing strength will result in illness. This illness might slowly become chronic and will lead to increased anxiety, which has a major impact on your body, and the final outcome might be an incurable disease.

Children must be taught that the only way towards happiness is learning how to live according to the Creator's will.

Reaching sainthood is every person's raison d'etre, and there is no purpose other than this from the moment of our birth. The word "Saint" suggests the union with God. God's love is boundless, and when we love Him and have unshakable faith, then we will become one with Him.

An old man once gave this advice to a village boy, who was ready to immigrate to the city: "You are about to travel on a great and dangerous ocean, my child." "I know," the child answered and added, after taking his small bible and a picture of the Virgin Mary from his pocket, "but I have a compass that will point me to the right path. My mother gave it to me."

This child grew up to be Georgios Rizaris, one greatest benefactors of Hellas.

The effects of prayer require godly action, which can't be measured scientifically. There are statistical studies, though, which demonstrate the positive influence of prayer. Those studies don't deal with the real kind of prayer, but with the superficial one. Dr. Randolph Byrd, a cardiologist from San Francisco, U.S.A mentions in a study he published at the Southern Medical Journal that patients who prayed reacted more positively to treatment, when they had to be admitted to the Coronary Care Unit, as far as their need for medication and respiratory assistance were concerned.

In 1996, only three medical hospitals taught spiritual medical care. Three years later, their number had increased to forty, and it keeps increasing.

Hellenic people have the good fortune of not needing such studies, as there are many examples of Saints, martyrs and even modern priests, who stood by their side during personal and national struggles.

We have a variety of examples from miracles of faith, either by direct invocation of God, Jesus Christ, the Virgin Mary, Saints, or by the mediation of a priest, a monk or an ascetic. Everyone has had some personal experience or even indirectly through friends who have come in contact with living Saints; people dedicated to God, who serve divine justice, can read your thoughts, look into your body and soul, predict the future, describe places they have never visited, know everything about people they have never met, give medical diagnosis and treatments; they are seen in different places at the same time, consider themselves to be the biggest sinners, radiate simplicity and humbleness, and stay away from the public eye.

Saint Nectarios, Saint Paisios, Father Jacobs Tsalikis, Saint Porphyrios, Father Philotheos Zervakis, Father Cleopas, Father Epiphanios Theodoropoulos, Father Sophronios of Essex, Father Germanos Stavrovouniotis, Father Amphilochios Makris, Father Gabriel Dionysatis, Father Demetrios Gagastathis and Father Chariton are just some of the bright examples of this century; holy persons who were united with God.

There isn't a particular place where someone can become a saint. Take Saint Porphyrios for example. For many years, he was just the priest of the small church of the polyclinic in Athen's

Omonoia square. A place can change after a while; it gains a different energy. A nursery school, for example, gives off a different energy than a retirement home. Places like the Garden of the Virgin Mary (the Holy Mount of Athos) or the Meteora, have gained a different dynamic.

The first picture, the Earth's crucifixion, shows nature as it gives out a scream of salvation, and points to Jesus Christ as its Savior. Humans kill whales, which serve as the ocean biological cleaning system. They swallow huge quantities of water, clean it, and then flush it out through their blowholes. Jesus, as He appears in the picture, is surrounded by light, in contrast to the world, which is far away from Him and covered in blood. (Father Zouros).

If, for some reason, you don't resort to prayer, you have the second, though of smaller value, option of using relaxation techniques, such as meditation, contemplation, eye movements and self-hypnosis. Muscles and tissues relax with these techniques, and the mind, at best, empties temporarily from thoughts and rests.

Meditation

Meditation means complete absence of conscious thought, whereas in prayer our thoughts have to be focused on our Heavenly Lord, Jesus Christ, the Virgin Mary, or the Saints.

The position of the seated Buddha, who sits still with his back straight, his legs crossed and his eyes closed, is the classic position of the meditating person. Perhaps it would be easier if the meditating person sat on a low stool or a fat pillow. It is said that Buddha sat meditating for six whole days and reached enlightenment.

It is difficult to keep your mind blank, even for a second. It takes hours of practice for someone to achieve it. The great meditators-

gurus, who "dedicate" their lives to eastern traditions, are capable of emptying their mind of every thought for a few minutes. If someone manages to keep his mind blank for just a single second, they will be filled with happiness that they will remember for the rest of their lives.

The absence of fear, anger and sexual feelings are the requirements for properly meditating. Also, your stomach mustn't be full. Meditation needs to be done in a quiet environment, and is more effective between 3am to 5am; many times it can be combined with lighting scented candles. Many experienced meditators try to find places with calm vibrations, such as places where battles have never happened and blood hasn't been shed. The time dedicated to meditation differs from person to person, and it depends on their physical (physical stamina) and psychic (calmness) condition. Twenty minutes of a meditation attempt are usually enough.

At the beginning of meditation it's better to focus on the air that you breathe in through your nostrils, continues its way through the trachea, enters the lungs (bronchi) and slowly fills even the remotest of their parts (alveoli). When they get fully expanded, your attention turns to the air that slowly escapes following the opposite way.

Breathing correctly is the most important element in the conscious forms of relaxation apart from prayer (love towards God).

Contemplation

Contemplation is an offshoot of meditation. It is performed by sitting comfortably in a quiet environment, with your eyes closed, and taking deep, relaxed breaths, while the mind is allowed to focus on a calm predetermined or random thought. You can either direct your thoughts towards a peaceful place or give your mind the freedom to follow any emerging thoughts.

The peaceful place could be a safe, quiet lake surrounded by grass, where you can picture yourself sitting on top a beach towel. Flowers of all colors surround you and, a bit further away, there are some trees with green leaves growing on their branches, where birds sit. The weather is sunny, the sky a deep blue with some wispy clouds, just enough so that the sunlight doesn't bother you.

Focus all of your senses to this image, as if it is something you really experience. Feel a light, quiet and refreshing breeze caress your skin. Feast on the colors of nature, the flowers, the trees, the lake and the sky. Listen to the birds singing and the rustle of the leaves. Smell the scents coming from the flowers, the herbs, the trees and the lake; they waft through the clean air.

You can set the scenery of this peaceful place according to your preferences, with things that will be good for you and won't be the cause for bad memories and problems, real or imagined.

Here you can place any person from your loved ones, or someone else (e.g. a Saint or an ascetic), who could help you with the problem that troubles you. You must never forget, though, that everything you might experience here belongs in the realm of imagination.

Eye movements

They are recommended for simple, quick relaxation, or in order to free yourselves from anger or negative feelings towards a particular person, who might have harmed you in some way.

Constant anger or hatred causes increasingly bigger psychosomatic damage. The eyes of people are the windows to their soul. Quick eye movements open a small window to the soul from where a tortuous weight might be released.

Technique: Very fast and constant eye movements towards all

directions, right and left, up and down, diagonally and in circles, until you feel dizzy (for two or three minutes).

It's an easy relaxation technique that can even be done in the workplace, by hiding your face behind your hands. You might realize that the more stressed you are, the less quickly you are able to move your eyes.

By rapidly moving your eyes, you will slowly relax and achieve faster movements.

In case of torment, hatred and negative emotions, you should think about the person who has hurt you, when you are close to completing the eye movements.

By repeating them comes the realization that anger, hatred and all of the ugly feelings, which consciously or unconsciously overwhelm you, disappear and are replaced by indifference.

It is of vital importance that your soul is empty of negative emotions. The existence of anything negative is harmful and might lead to your collapse, just like wood collapses when it gets infected by woodworm.

It's obviously better if there are experienced persons present, so that the patient's eyes can follow their quick hand movements.

This technique is indispensable for those who work for many hours on a computer, spend a lot of time in front of a screen (e.g. television), or drive for many hours, especially at night. It is understandable that, in these cases, the eyes get tired, giving off a "burning" feeling and that this tiredness-burning spreads to the head and the rest of the body.

A three-minute break every one or two hours, so that you can calmly rotate your neck and apply the rapid eye movement technique, will improve your mood and give you relief from headaches, neck pain, anxiety, constant fatigue and sleepiness.

It is recommended to repeat these eye movements three times daily for treating anxiety.

Self-hypnosis

Lie down on your back or sit comfortably in a quiet, warm environment with one of your hands raised. Bend your hand to the elbow and raise it in a right angle with your elbow still resting on the bed or on the armchair. If this position seems confusing, then just freely stretch your hands on the bed's surface, or rest them comfortably on the arms of your armchair.

First stage of self-hypnosis: Focus your gaze on a point upwards, so that your eyes are turned towards your forehead (e.g. people with short hair could focus their gaze on the hair growing over their forehead). The most important thing of all is to keep your eyes still and, of course, not to move your body or speak. Observe the point-area you have chosen (it just needs to be a few centimeters long) for any color or texture irregularities. After thirty seconds, let your eyes focus exclusively on a small dot of this area. Take calm breaths. When you feel your eyes getting tired and your eyelids getting so heavy that you can't keep them open (in about two minutes), just let them close.

During those two minutes, alternate your attention between the senses of hearing and touch; focus on a slight sound-noise for a few seconds (small or large background can always be found everywhere) and then focus on a part of your body touching the bed or the armchair (e.g. hand, head, heel, elbow). This alternating should happen at least three times. Try not to blink when your eyes start feeling heavy. The eyelids should only close once, when your eyes have gotten really tired. Then, the second stage of self-hypnosis begins.

Second stage of self-hypnosis: As you lay with your eyes closed, keep your breath calm (deeply breathing in and out without forcing yourself) and mentally repeat: "every time I exhale, the more my hand will lower itself, the more I will relax." When your hand comes to rest on the bed or the armchair, you will be completely relaxed.

If you kept your hand down during the first stage of self-hypnosis, then in the second part you should repeat: "every time I exhale I will get more and more relaxed."

The third stage is optional and is about how to deepen your relaxation. The first possible way is by thinking of a number after every exhale, and mentally repeating: "the lower the number, the deeper my relaxation gets." Mentally count backwards from ten to one.

When you reach one, then you may start with auto suggestions: "I will be healthier with every day that passes by ...or more patient ...or calmer ...or better in sales ... or my immune system will get stronger ...or my knee will hurt less and less ...or I will eat less food ...or I will smoke less ...or drink less alcohol ...I will not get an allergic reaction by eating this food..."

You may go down an imaginary staircase (you step even deeper into relaxation) and find yourself in that peaceful place described in the contemplation part. There you can ask for help or get even deeper into relaxation.

Fourth and final stage of self-hypnosis: Ending deep relaxation, or self-hypnosis, is achieved by mentally counting from five to one and saying: "Five. My eyes feel refreshed by this cool, crystal clear running mountain water." (Exhale.) "Four. My whole body is refreshed and relaxed." (Exhale.) "Three. I will be more relaxed and healthier with every day that passes by." (Exhale.) "Two. My eyes are refreshed, my body is renewed, I feel wonderful, and I'm ready to open my eyes." After the next exhalation, mentally count to the last number, which is one, and open your eyes right away feeling truly renewed.

You have to keep in mind that you might try any auto-suggestion you wish, but there is no guarantee that your wish-suggestion will become true. Deep relaxation, though, is a prerequisite.

After the self-hypnosis session, carefully try to check, with all the necessary precautions, if your suggestion worked.

In case of mental or psychological disorder, a psychiatrist should be consulted before attempting any self-hypnosis.

SECTION 2: DIET

Ancient Hellenic and Chinese theory

Food and the air we breathe, assisted by the gene substrate (heredity), mental stability and physical exercise, are the basic elements for the constant creation, function and regeneration of the human body's cells and tissues, leading to physical and mental well-being.

The importance of nutrition in maintaining good (primarily physical) health, and in the prevention and treatment of illnesses is therefore recognized.

Hippocrates (c.460-c.377 BC), who is considered to be the father of modern medicine, is quoted as saying "let your food be your medicine, and medicine be your food."

According to the Empedoclean-Hippocratic doctrine, humans and food are categorized in four types, depending on their temperature and moisture.

The phlegmatic types have a cool and moist body; selfish and cold-blooded, they suffer from respiratory viruses (and can easily develop pharyngitis or bronchitis) and stomach ailments (burping and indigestion).

The melancholic types have a cool and dry body; depressive and cold-blooded, they are known for their bouts of depressions and indigestion (their bowels are a still bog).

The choleric types have a warm and dry body; they are usually intolerant of heat, especially when it's not accompanied by humidity. Not only does their fiery temperament cause friction in their relationships with their loved ones, but also hepatic disorders and problems with their ligaments-tendons and genitalia.

The sanguine types have a warm and moist body; they are optimists with a high blood count (note that smokers have a high blood count, but few of them are sanguine types) and a round, florid face. Humid, hot weather makes them feel uncomfortable. They usually suffer from urinary tract infections, hypochondria, mild anxiety and slight obesity. Still, they are good-hearted and with a friendly disposition.

These characteristics are not present in every type, due to the ever present biodiversity.

The much-desired balance can be achieved by knowing your type (phlegmatic, melancholic, choleric or sanguine), eating food, and drinking herbal teas of the opposite temperature and moistness.

Cool types of food: fish, lemons, barley, vinegar, lentils, fava beans, hard-boiled eggs, most kinds of fruit, vegetables, and herbs, along with most kinds of dairy products.

Warm types of food: meat, wheat, salt, pepper, sweets, fatty food, honey, mature cheese, olive oil, basil, rocket leaves, cress, garlic, onions, celery, radish, asparagus; fruit, such as sweet grapes, apples (not crab apples), figs, pomegranates, melons; nuts, such as almonds, walnuts and chestnuts.

Dry types of food: salt, vinegar, dried fava beans, rice, chestnuts, walnuts and barley.

Moist types of food: lettuce, peaches, apricots, cherries, fish, apples, fresh fava beans.

But how can you discover the type you belong to? It's difficult, and that's why this doctrine only has a small following. A somewhat simple way is the muscle test for selecting food-substances,

p. 30, where after choosing one of the four food categories that suits you best, you know you have the opposite temperament.

Every type has grades. For example: a first grade sanguine type is more balanced than a third grade type of the same category.

Food also has subcategories. This is why Hippocrates, for example, would call a food or herb, 1st, 2nd, 3rd degree moist, and advises people accordingly.

A healthy body should be everyone's goal from childhood, because "prevention is better than the cure".

What dietary habits should children have, and how much should adults change theirs so that they can live longer and enjoy a better quality of life?

The ancient Hellenes used to say "all in good measure", but how can food quantity and quality be measured?

The food portions should be such that you leave the table still slightly hungry without a bloated or heavy stomach. Eat only when you are really hungry and don't use food as a way to deal with anxiety, eating anything within reach, or in the fridge. Keep in mind that most of the times you are thirstier than hungry, and that, by drinking 2 litres of water daily, it is possible to cover the recommended water intake and eat less at the same time.

Eating little, combined with physical exercise and mental balance, must be our battle cry in the fight against the damage caused by the passing of time. You should eat to live and not live to eat.

Overeating translates to obesity or increased toxins concentration because, in this modern industrial age, food, water and air have lost their purity. The only thing that differs is the amount of toxins in each of them.

Obesity is a plague for many developed countries, where fast food, anxiety, sedentary work that lasts many hours and lack of physical exercise reign supreme.

Medical doctors are aware that obesity is usually accompanied by many illnesses such as hypertension, diabetes, cardiovascular diseases, hip and knee osteoarthritis, and spondylarthropathies.

Even if overeating doesn't cause weight gain, the body is still burdened with a high degree of toxins leading to the appearance of acute or chronic diseases.

Unfortunately, the food you eat isn't pure, so your defense must be eating less.

One only needs to remember the Chernobyl disaster, where radiation leaked from the city's nuclear power plant, polluting the air and the ground; the "mad cow" disease scare in the UK; the Belgian poultry meat contaminated with dioxin; the 43 tones of GMO rice confiscated by the Hellenic commission of food quality control in November 2006; the mineral-oil contaminated sunflower oil, which was used in a wide range of products (May 2008).

Scientists keep giving warnings about the consequences of groundwater contamination by pesticides, insecticides, fertilizers and waste, which are some of the toxins that find their way into the food chain.

Another serious issue is that the public is uninformed of the short and long-term consequences that the accumulation of food toxins will have in consumers' health. Even though food toxins are harmless in small quantities, they might be harmful when overaccumulated or combined with other substances and chemical compounds.

The rule of moderation, which Ancient Hellenes revered, should exist in every aspect of your life. There should be moderation in both quantity and quality in food categories.

Chinese people categorize food according to its taste, which they regard as its quintessence. According to the Chinese worldview, everything is divided into yin and yang aspects, though they both co-exist. Nothing in this world is 100 per cent yin or yang.

It is usual to consume only yang food, such as sweet, salty, and spicy, and very few of the yin food categories, such as sour and bitter food (aubergines, artichokes, radishes, rocket, bitter almonds, some types of olives, grape fruit, common sage, chamomile tea, coffee, bitter chocolate). There should be a balance between flavors and yin-yang in your meals.

Overindulgence of yang food has turned people into victims of numerous illnesses (diabetes mellitus, vasculopathy, coronary artery disease, high blood pressure, lumbar disk disease, osteoporosis, kidney failure, etc.), including tooth decay.

According to recent data from the Hellenic Orthodontic Society (2005), every adult has been affected by tooth decay. Only 3.3 per cent have healthy gums between the age of 35 and 44, while 40 per cent have lost all of their natural teeth between the age of 65 and 74.

Most people have yang characters; they are stressed, impatient, and irritable with exaggerated emotional responses, hasty, too busy, and easily plagued by insomnia. That's why they need yin food.

People with yin characters are calm, lethargic and feel uncomfortable in cold weather; they have cold limbs, restrain their emotional responses, are prone to depression, and need yang food.

Yin and yang always coexist, and people's characters contain elements from both categories.

Yin food: Vegetables, fruit (apart from bananas and melons), whole grains (rice, wheat, oats, rye, barley, corn, millet), sprouts, seeds, olive oil, yoghurt, pasta, angel hair pasta (capellini), bread, milk, most herbs (with the more characteristic representative being chamomile), boiled and steamed food.

Yin food is generally light, easily digestible, and preferable to the average city inhabitants, who need calmness, but also strength and energy.

Yang food: meat, fish, eggs, pulses, olives, fat, butter, cheese, pastries, honey, some herbs (e.g. ironwort), coffee, sauces, alcohol (the higher the ethanol content is, the more yang it is), sugar, salt, chocolate, canned food, spices, GMOs, smoked, fried and grilled food.

Yang food has many calories and they overburden the gastrointestinal system during their digestion.

Food portions are also of great significance. The bigger, or the more processed the food portions, the more yang they are.

The easily digestible kinds of food are yin, the less easily digestible ones, which make the stomach feel heavy, are yang.

The yin food is transformed into yang food after being processed or having other kinds of food added to it.

Examples of food that has been turned from yin to yang are:

Bitter chocolate (yin) in which sugar is added by the "sweet" industries and, strictly speaking, turns into yang food.

Sage tea (yin) turns into yang if honey or sugar is added in it.

Vegetables, fruit, animals raised with the use of chemicals, antibiotics and pesticides are turned from yin to yang or become more yang.

The off season production of fruit, vegetable, or other food turns them into yang. They are usually a result of violating nature, which as a chain reaction negatively affect people.

Nutritional balance is achieved only when there is a preference for pure, unprocessed, certified organic products.

Many people rightly believe that "you are what you eat and what you think", your genealogical tree, of course, plays a part, too. When you eat meat all the time, you also consume the animal's agony while it was being slaughtered, and the toxins produced at the moment of its death. As a result, you receive aggressiveness and tension, in contrast to the consumption of pasta (flour-cereal produce), which results in the intake of calm earthly energy.

Folk wisdom advises that local products are the best. People should eat local products, which nature provides them with. When they have no respect for nature, they will pay for it, sooner or later. Besides, earth's natural resources should be wisely used. Just imagine how much fuel is needed to transport food products from all over the world in your country, and, correspondingly, how much the planet gets polluted. Everyone must be environmentally conscious.

People's way of life is as important as the area they live in. People living in cities are part of a sedentary lifestyle, and that's why they need simple yin food. If they live in cold climates (or during the cold winter months) or if they have menial jobs, they need warm food, rich in calories, such as pulses, rice, soups, eggs, cheese and meet.

You should always prefer seasonal and organic, if possible, food products.

Muscle test for selecting food-substances

Muscle testing is a simple way that allows you to find if a food item, substance, herb, or herb combination is suitable for you or not, if it would improve your health or not.

Two persons are needed, the tester and the examiner. At first, the tester must drink two glasses of water and then extend both hands before clasping them together. The examiner places both palms on the tester's wrists and tries for a few seconds to lower the tester's arms, without using too much force, though, image 5. It isn't a strength contest. Naturally, the tester's arms should resist the force from the examiner's hands and keep both arms raised.

Then, the tester picks up a food item-substance with the dominant hand and extends only that hand, while clutching the food item. The examiner places a palm on the tester's wrist and exerts the same restrained force as before.

If the stretched arm is lowered, then the food item-substance is not suitable for the tester. If it isn't, then the food item-substance is suitable for the tester. A food item-substance, or one of its ingredients, might not be healthy, pure, or is something downright harmful for the tester. If you have intolerance of a food item-substance, or if you are allergic to it, then your arm will get lowered.

The same test can be repeated with various food items-substances. It will become obvious that sometimes your hand completely loses its strength and your arm is lowered pretty easily, while others it will hardly get lowered or it won't be forced down at all. This happens because some food items-substances are not suitable for you at all or some of them might only be slightly or truly suitable for you,

The muscle testing can be done while using either hand or both hands at the same time. After a few times, the tester's hands will become tired, at which point the testing should stop until the tester is fully rested.

Both initial (without the food item-substance) and final testing (with the food item-substance) should be done at the same spot (place). No electrical appliances should be turned on between the two tests. Both the tester and the examiner must have neutral thoughts for the food item-substance, which is about to be tested.

But what if it's about a small child or a baby, who can't participate in the testing? In this case, three persons are needed: the child, the tester and the examiner. Let's suppose that the mother is the tester, and the father acts as the examiner. The mother stretches her dominant hand and places the other over the child's belly button. The father exerts restrained force for a couple of seconds on the mother's wrist, so that her hand can remain in the same position. The same procedure is followed for the final testing, with the difference that the mother holds the food item-substance in her dominant hand. If the mother's hand doesn't fall, then food item-substance is suitable for the child. If the opposite happens, it is unsuitable for the child.

If you find food products-substances, which are unsuitable for you, verify the testing with an experienced examiner. If you find it impossible, avoid eating that food or using those substances for a while, in order to see if you feel better.

The same testing can be applied to find out which herb, or which part of a plant (root, leaves, stem, nuts, blossoms) and what dosage is suitable for you. Still, show caution and always try to listen to your body. Your senses will not let you down.

Reviewing the testing: if you put some laundry soap in a plastic or paper bag and follow the muscle testing for selecting food-substances, then your hand should drop, otherwise the testing hasn't been applied correctly.

Simple Advice

Eat small portions of local organic products. The less you eat, the more chances you have of living a longer life with fewer problems.

Concentrate on what you eat during mealtimes and feel gratitude towards the Creator for everything that nature generously offers. That means no television and lively discussions while eating.

Avoid drinking water during mealtimes because water passes very quickly through the stomach and carries away food that needs more time in the stomach and contact with its acidic liquids in order to be properly digested.

Fruit should be consumed before and not after meals. You can start your meal after half an hour, the time usually needed for their digestion.

Since some nutrients take longer to digest, fruit should be eaten before meals or after four hours, in between meals.

Food, especially starchy food (bread, potatoes, rice, pasta), should be chewed very well, as they have to be mixed with saliva in order to be digested.

Finely chopped, and particularly mashed, food is more easily digested. When patients go back to their regular diet, they should start by eating mushed, easily digested food (e.g. pureed boiled zucchinis and carrots).

Eat slowly, so as not to overtax your gastrointestinal system with indigestible food and give your body time to feel full.

Avoid mixing many kinds of food during meals. This may lead to a heavy stomach, which slows down digestion's natural process, and food becomes a cause for energy loss instead of gain.

A good trick for eating less is drinking two glasses of water before every meal. This will make you feel fuller while eating a smaller amount of food.

You should drink plenty of water daily; at least eight glasses. Water helps the kidneys function normally. The more sweet or salty things you eat, the more water you need.

Since everything in medicine is individualized, you should listen to your body's advice on which kinds of food, in which quantities, and in which combinations suit you best. The best medical doctor is yourself. This is who you should listen to.

You should avoid lying down directly after a meal. It would be better if you did some light housework or took a short walk.

The above mentioned should be applied on a daily basis for precautionary medical reasons.

In case of an illness or intoxication, the raw food diet (eating seeds, herbs and fruit), the fruit therapy or the fasting therapy should be followed.

However a physician with experience in these treatments may advise you against the above mentioned therapies for specific reasons, such as: low blood pressure and weakness of the organism caused by fasting or dieting.

Raw Food Diet

Heating-grilling gives yang characteristics to food. That's why TCM doctors recommend the raw food diet, which means yin food (it hasn't undergone yang conversion), to patients with yang characters or mild yang diseases. They also recommend hot meat soups to frail patients whose illness is yin in nature and relates to the harmful effects of cold weather.

There are many health conscious people who argue that cooking food alters it to such a degree that it becomes harmful to the body. They suggest eating raw foods in their natural state.

Seeds, herbs, vegetables, fruit and nuts, uncooked and unsalted are all included in the raw food diet.

It is the simplest detoxifying treatment, which can be combined with the fasting periods of the Orthodox Christian tradition.

Higher church leaders, being aware of people's tendency to overeat, but also of fasting's therapeutic effect both on the spirit (humility and discipline), and on the body, established periods of refraining from consuming animal products: Lent, from Pure Monday to Easter Sunday; from 1st August to 15th August, the Christmas period from 15th November to 25th December, as well as every Wednesday and Friday.

Christian fasting, of course, mainly aims at spiritual fasting, as what comes out of one's mouth (words and deeds) is more harmful than what one eats.

Nowadays, and particularly in developed countries, the vast majority of diseases are yang in nature, so raw food diet and other detoxifying treatments (fruit therapy and fasting therapy) can definitely be implemented.

Almond milk

Many people will wonder if it's possible to live without meat and regular milk. It is possible to use almond milky extract, instead of cow, sheep or goat milk. Take a large handful of almonds and boil them in water for a couple of minutes (so that it will be easier to remove their skin). After removing their skin, put them in the blender, where you can also add some orange juice and a small quantity of parsley leaves. The resulting thick liquid is strained through a fine sieve, a cheesecloth or a tulle. This way the solid small almond pieces are separated from the white almond extract (milk).

Almond milk has been used in the rearing of many children, who were allergic to animal milk, or their mothers were unable to breastfeed them. There is also soya milk, but since there is the possibility of GMO soya, and since everybody can produce their own almond milk and be sure of its purity, then you come to the realization that almond milk is the best choice.

You shouldn't be concerned over not receiving animal proteins, even for a limited time. The theory of essential amino acids being found only in animal products has long since been refuted. You can get all the essential amino acids that make up proteins by eating a variety of food, such as nuts, fruit and vegetables. This is incontestably proven by the thousands of people who have been exclusively vegetarians from a very young age.

Be careful so that there aren't any bitter almonds mixed together with the regular ones. You shouldn't eat more than eight bitter almonds (and less than 8 for children, and none at all for infants) a day because there is a serious risk of getting cyanide poisoning.

Sprouts

The word "sprout" is unknown to many people, but you will have to get used to them and make them a part of your daily diet. Sprouts are seeds that have germinated into very young plants. Their nutritional value is immeasurable because, when it germinates, the seed is just like a pregnant mother, who gives the best nutrients, minerals, vitamins, enzymes and abundant energy to her child.

How to make sprouts: Fill the bottom of a water glass with raw lentils up to three centimetres in height. Fill it with water and leave it there for eight hours or overnight. Then, pour the water out, fill it again with water, and pour the water out again. Place a paper towel (or cloth) over the mouth of the glass and secure it with a rubber band. This way you have achieved the humid condition the lentils should be in. Change the water every six to seven hours.

In two or three days, the lentils should have sprouted, and when the sprouts size is equal to that of the seed, then remove the lentils from the glass and place them on a cloth to dry. When dry, you can put them in a jar and store them in the refrigerator. You can eat as many lentils as you want directly from the jar with a spoon or put them in a salad or in your food.

If the seeds haven't germinated within three days, it means that they are of low quality, so discard them. The sooner they germinate the better quality they are.

You can put seeds in a pan with soil and cover them with a little more soil. If you pour some water over them once in a while, they will germinate. When they have reached a height of 10 centimetres, you can cut the sprouts with scissors (don't uproot them) and eat them in a salad. This way, not only is your diet enriched with very beneficial ingredients, but you also have a weapon against expensiveness, and hunger (in times of food shortage) because the sprouts will grow back.

I highly recommend sprouts for treating anemia, debility, fatigue, and as preventative measure, since it is a multivitamin food.

Image 30 shows lentil sprouts and wheat in the glass.

Caution: if you are allergic to any type of seed, try to desensitize yourself using all the knowledge contained in this book.

Fruit Therapy

This treatment means that you only eat a certain kind of fruit and have as much water as you want. Even coffee and chewing gums are prohibited. I recommend the consumption of a single kind of fruit as treatment and detoxification, in contrast to eating many kinds of fruit.

The grape diet (the grape is regarded as the king of fruit) and the orange diet (orange is regarded as the queen of fruit) are the most prevalent fruit therapies, but one can also follow the apple diet or the watermelon diet, or use other fruit, such as tangerines and pears.

It is more effective to drink freshly squeezed juice from the particular fruit and plenty glasses of water in the in-between. If, instead of drinking their juice, you eat the raw fruit, you will be hungrier, because, on the one hand more gastric liquids will be secreted and on the other you will need more energy to digest the raw fruit.

The secret of the fruit therapy is to get out gastrointestinal system used to eating a particular, very easily digestible type of food (fruit), so that the energy used for digestion is minimal, and plenty of our physical energy is directed into the affected system, organ or tissue. The human organism with its large self healing potential (remember that people have been created in the image and likeness of God) will direct its energy to the right target with surprisingly good results.

The way patients will return to their normal diet is hugely significant. If someone underwent a ten-day fruit juice therapy, then it will take them five days of gradual return to a normal diet. If someone underwent a ten-day fruit therapy by eating the fruit, and not drinking its juice, three days will be required for their gradually return to a normal diet. If after the end of the fruit therapy you instantly go back to eating regular food, especially indigestible kinds of food, such as steak, brassica olarecea (cabbage, broccoli, cauliflower etc.) or bean soup, then you may end up in hospital with a perforated stomach.

In the case of fruit juice therapy, one should return to their normal diet by eating small portions of the following daily meals, morning and evening, in order of ease of digestion. We start from the more easily digestible and continue to the most difficult to digest.

Initial meals: thin vermicelli soup (with olive oil and lemon) or, for a fruit therapy that lasted for few days, boiled zucchini and carrots (with a lemon and olive oil dressing).

Later meals:

Thick pasta soup (with baby pasta stars, or couscous) or boiled orzo with tomato.

Well-boiled unrefined rice with yogurt and raw tomato or boiled mixed frozen vegetables, (during the afternoon) local raw fruit (no bananas or melons) or wholemeal bread with tomato, feta cheese and uncooked, unsalted nuts.

Before going back to your regular diet:

Spaghetti with tomato sauce and a piece of fruit (during the afternoon), or a light burger with salad and a piece fruit in the afternoon, in case of fruit therapy for a few days.

In case you follow a six-day fruit juice therapy:

On the seventh day: eat boiled zucchini and carrots (for lunch and dinner).

On the eighth day: orzo cooked with tomato sauce.

On the ninth day: boiled mixed frozen vegetables with a little wholemeal bread and local fresh fruit (no bananas or melons) during the afternoon.

On the 10th day: You can eat normally.

In case you follow a six-day pure fruit therapy:

On the seventh day: orzo with tomato sauce (for lunch and dinner)

On the eighth: boiled mixed frozen vegetables with a little wholemeal bread and local fresh fruit (no banana or melon) in the afternoon.

While you gradually return to your normal diet, you should eat small portions, thoroughly chew the food, and stop eating before your stomach starts feeling heavy. If it does, stop eating. On the following day, have the same kind of meal.

When fruit therapy or fasting therapy are properly applied, but you haven't been cured, then, in many cases, excessive anxiety is to blame along with emotional tension and thoughts that cause mental and cognitive imbalance; as a consequence, there is the manifestation of physical illness.

People relax and begin to think differently after detoxifying themselves. As an example, I will mention the ascetics, who reach high spiritual levels not only by holding a continuous, constant inner prayer, but by also undergoing continuous fasts, which require eating a few simple kinds of food or not eating at all.

Answers to some usual questions patients might ask their medical doctor:

Will I get hungry? During the first three days, there will be a slight feeling of hunger, but by drinking enough water or by using acupuncture, the patient will feel satiated.

During the following days, the patient doesn't feel hungry at all, and may even cook for others or even accompany them to the most abundant meals, since the amount of gastric acids secreted are just enough to digest the fruit (when normally all you need to do is see or talk about food, and your stomach starts secreting gastric acids).

Will I be able to work normally? Yes. The only problem someone might face is orthostatic hypotension. So, it would be advisable to avoid suddenly getting up when you have been in a lying or sitting position beforehand (e.g. to answer the phone), and certainly avoid working in high places or do heavy manual labor or some other type of work, where dizziness you might experience can be dangerous to you and those around you. In general, though, it's a regiment that can be followed by a working person.

How long can someone live on just drinking the same natural, freshly squeezed fruit juice? People with no hypotension or stomach problems, which would be adversely affected by the particular fruit, can follow the fruit therapy for up to four days. If you are going to follow it for a larger number of days, then you must be under the supervision of a qualified physician. People can survive on just drinking the same fruit juice for four months, but only if their condition improves, and only under medical supervision.

For what diseases is it suitable? In order to answer this question, the causes of the disease should be known. Unfortunately, despite the progress of science, the majority of diseases are of unknown cause and, usually, there are multifactor causes involved.

When the main cause of a disease is overeating or eating harmful types of food, the fruit therapy, the fasting therapy, and the raw food diet play a central role in the treatment.

When the main cause is anxiety, fear, anger, or other negative emotions, then the self-restraint that patients are required to demonstrate during these treatments is the first step towards being cured. The second step is relaxation, which is helpful towards changing their way of thinking and their reactions towards external stimuli.

Most people in developed countries overburden their stomachs and they are accustomed to overeating, which results in a built-up of toxins in their organisms, since there is no kind of food that is pure nowadays.

It is widely known that air pollution is caused by motor vehicles, heating, factories, nuclear accidents, wars, etc. Everybody has begun to realize the ramifications of the aquifer contamination. We all know that the over-production of livestock, poultry and fish, in farms, fields and in greenhouses, is aided by the use of substances often harmful to humans.

It is also common knowledge that everyone has been eating GMO food products, but their type and quantities are unknown.

It is an unpleasant fact that DDT (i.e. notorious insecticide that was widely used a few decades ago) has been found in the fat deposits of Antarctica's penguins.

People ingest toxins through their food, inhale them with breathing, and absorb them through their skin. Selfishness, fear, materialistic desires, vanity, the everyday emotional tensions at work, in relationships, and in child-rearing, add an incalculable number of mental toxins.

Our cells and intercellular spaces have become a place of garbage- toxins disposal, to the pleasure of various diseases.

You should decide to only eat small portions of pure foods and follow detoxifying treatments, so that you eat the least amount of toxins possible and then you are able to expel or disable them. Detoxification is good for almost all physical and mental illnesses.

If a patient with a low body weight suffers from a lot of stress, then the physician's first care should be to help the patient with alternative forms of medicine (e.g. thermal baths, acupuncture), the second should be to advise the patient about different relaxation methods, the third should be to recommend eating healthier foods, and the fourth should be to advise the patient to review their lifestyle.

If overweight patients have anxiety problems, the physician should introduce the options of detoxifying treatments, relaxation techniques, alternative forms of medicine, changing eating habits and lifestyle.

If normal weight patients deal with normal stress issues, then the physician should recommend alternative forms of medicine, methods of relaxation and short detoxifying treatments (raw food diet, fruit therapy). The patient should also attempt to find the causes of the disease.

The patient who is following a non-pharmacological alternative medical treatment and is not improving or is getting worse should change treatment or turn to traditional pharmaceutical medicine. It should also be noted that when a major illness which usually requires hospitalization is involved, then the first action to be taken should be medication or surgical treatment. It is vital that patients monitor their health's progress by recording or remembering their pre-treatment clinical image and realize whether it has improved or has remained stable–stagnant, or if it has worsened. Patients must show trust in the regular use of diagnostic imaging and blood tests, which will make them more confident in following their treatment.

Fasting Therapy

In the non-pharmacological medical terminology, fasting therapy or just fasting, means that patients drink only water and aren't consuming food or chewing gum or using toothpaste to clean their teeth (i.e. they brush their teeth with a plain toothbrush) or drinking hot beverages or smoking.

The rationale of this therapy is that the deprivation of food-energy will initially destroy the abnormal cells and then stop the abnormal functions. Healthy cells (i.e. because they are healthy) and basic healthy functions will withstand the energy deprivation and will survive because the human body is fashioned with wisdom.

For a relatively large time frame, your body will not be starved off vitamins, minerals, proteins, carbohydrates or anything else. You have to realize that you have huge energy deposits.

When dogs get sick, they stop eating altogether and just sit in a sheltered corner. Even if food is placed near them, they won't touch it, only surviving by drinking water. When they start eating again, you can say that the dog has been cured. Dogs understand without any guidance when the abnormal cells have been destroyed, and, therefore, they resume eating, in order to provide their normal cells with energy and strength.

After observing this, the same treatment could be applied to humans. This treatment should always be done under the guidance and supervision of a physician trained in this kind of treatment. It would be advisable for patients to undergo a full medical checkup (i.e. complete blood count, levels of glucose, urea, creatinine, transaminase, potassium, sodium, urine analysis, erythrocyte sedimentation rate) before starting their fasting, because, if they undergo the same medical tests during the course of the treatment, they will be able to have comparative data and determine their organs' proper function or failure.

Keep in mind that fasting should be done under medical supervision and certainly not by patients who are starving or are continuously malnourished.

Once you take the decision to follow this treatment, you just have to wake up in the morning and avoid eating. Gradually stopping your food intake isn't recommended. In the early days of the treatment, you will have bad breath, your tongue will have a thick pale yellow coating on top, and your morning urine will be dark yellow. The yellow tongue coating, which will progressively become lighter in color, can be removed daily by using a soft toothbrush.

At the beginning of the fasting therapy you might feel debilitation of your strength because your body unlearns its habits and is trying to adjust to the food deprivation. If you feel weak, then rest, get some sleep and drink extra water. If you still can't handle the weakness, acupuncture will help you during the first few days.

A normal weight patient should drink at least eight glasses of water (i.e. two litres) daily, and this amount should be increased by a glass of water for every ten extra kilograms. Patients should be aware of the fact that a large part of the eliminated toxins will be expelled from their body through urine. Drinking large quantities of water is required, so that the renal function is not disturbed by the existence of a large amount of gathered toxins.

After the first five days, your body has gotten used to fasting, and you feel almost normal. There is no feeling of hunger, though you might have the urge to complain (e.g. why do others get to eat, and not me). Fecal excretion stops. You might defecate once or twice in the first twenty days of fasting, but you might defecate even after forty days, although you are not eating, which indicates how many useless things there are in your intestine. There is no need to have enemas done, in order to quickly get rid of the junk in your bowels. Let nature take action.

While you fast, you should exercise very mildly and not do heavy manual labor.

During fasting, patients should gradually improve. There should be less subjective complaints, and better objective findings, (i.e. through laboratory and imaging tests). If there is no improvement, then the supervising physician should reconsider on whether the fasting therapy is the right treatment for the particular patient.

Once the patient is completely cured, the first morning urine (i.e. before drinking water in the morning, and after eight hours have passed since the last time you drank some) is clear in color, the tongue is bright red (i.e. like a baby's) and most importantly, the patient wants to eat. Then, the fasting therapy is completed, and the patient should gradually return to normal eating habits.

If the patient that has fasted for many days wants to eat (i.e. has the appetite to eat, and has asked for food), then, regardless of whether the illness has been cured or not, the physician should allow the patient to begin the gradual return to a regular diet.

But, for how long can one live only on water? The IRA prisoners, who went on hunger strike in the 1980's, while they were incarcerated in British prisons, died after 45 days of fasting (having been through enormous emotional upheavals and living in a subhuman environment, with dampness, etc.). The famous world record for longer fasting is 119 days. One can survive only on water while living in a familiar environment (or a specialized clinic) under medical supervision for several weeks. I have personally supervised a young female patient, who fasted for 63 days, and a young male patient who fasted for 50 days.

The way patients will return to their normal diet is of huge significance. It is a thousand times better to undergo fewer days of detoxification and slowly return to a normal diet, than to try and undergo a larger period of fasting or fruit therapy, and then skip some of the days of gradual re-introduction to normal food intake. If, after several days of fasting, you eat an indigestible food (e.g. burgers), you may even die. This is what happened to several starving (frightfully malnourished) Jewish prisoners of German concentration camps. After they were freed, they ate more than they should have and died because of this sudden overeating.

A return to normal eating habits should be very gradual, and food should be eaten in small quantities. You can start with thin vermicelli soups (without any oil, salt, or other additional ingredients), drinking only the liquid.

In the following days you may drink some orange juice, gradually increasing the quantity, and then eat the entire thin vermicelli soup.

As more days pass, you can add small quantities of the following foods which you should increase gradually:

Mashed boiled zucchini, and pureed boiled zucchini with carrots, first plain and then with a lemon-olive oil dressing in your diet.

Later you can gradually add celery (apium graveolens) and some potatoes, boiling them together and eating them pureed.

Boiled, non-pureed, zucchini with lemon-olive oil dressing, and then soft-boiled carrots.

Thick pasta soup (with pasta stars or couscous).

Plain tomato salad with boiled zucchini and carrots and lemon-oil dressing.

Then, the following dishes are recommended (as daily midday-evening meals) in the following order:

Orzo with tomato paste.

Risotto with sheep milk yoghurt.

Boiled frozen mixed vegetables.

Boiled green beans with unrefined rice.

Wholemeal bread with tomato and feta.

Yoghurt raisins and uncooked, unsalted nuts, such as almonds, walnuts, peanuts, and seasonal fruit.

Poached eggs with tomato salad (with oregano and feta), and wholemeal bread.

Thin noodles with tomato sauce.

Chicken soup with chunks of chicken.

Fish soup with chunks of fish.

Light meatloaf with a tomato-cucumber salad.

Lettuce and chicken breast salad.

Finally add meat, pulses, wild cabbage, onions, garlic, spinach, and generally heavy, indigestible foods.

The fasting therapy and the return to a normal eating pattern should both last the same number of days. So, if you fasted for ten days, you need ten more days for a gradual return to your regular diet with the help of the above mentioned easily digestible meals (vermicelli soup, orange juice, angel hair, mashed, boiled zucchini, baby pasta, orzo, yogurt risotto, boiled mixed frozen vegetables, wholemeal bread with a raw tomato etc.).

Those who have undergone the fruit therapy or the fasting therapy realize the true value of a single orange, and how many months of effort, with a lot of help from the soil, the sun and the weather conditions, an orange tree needs in order to produce this single piece of fruit.

They realize that their thoughts become simpler and not only do they perceive the divine action in the creation of an orange, but also the existence of the vast internal energy that God has gifted to humans.

Through abstinence by fasting or following fruit therapy, people mold not only their body, but their spirit, as well.

Mediterranean Diet

The Mediterranean diet is rich in fresh fruit, fresh vegetables, pulses, olive oil, olives, uncooked-unsalted nuts, and whole grains. It also includes fish, a little meat and small quantities of wine (usually red).

The Mediterranean diet doesn't include many dairy products, animal products (especially red meat), processed-refined products, sugar or alcohol. It is rich in vegetable oils, fiber, antioxidants and free radical neutralizers.

The result is low cholesterol and triglyceride levels, high unsaturated fatty acid levels, and maintaining a normal body weight in old age. Of course, one should not lose sight of the fact that this diet was and should stay connected to eating less. Small food portions are the key element of the Mediterranean diet.

Over the last 25 years, all medical studies link the Mediterranean diet to protection against cardiovascular diseases and longevity.

It protects the lung, the brain and lowers the risk of serious lung diseases, such as emphysema and bronchitis.

People who followed a mostly Mediterranean diet were 68 per cent less likely to develop Alzheimer's disease than people with quite different eating patterns. It lowers the risk of diabetes mellitus, hypertension, arthritis, kidney and gall stones, and cancer.

During childhood, it protects against the symptoms of asthma and nasal allergies.

Genetically Modified Organisms or GMOs

Mutated types of food have been cunningly renamed genetically modified, because the word "mutated" sounds very heavy and unattractive to consumers.

What is genetically modified food? The products of mutated organisms, which are served in your plate.

Genetically modified organisms, or GMOs, are produced in laboratories with the help of genetic engineering.

Their production process includes the extraction of selected genes from one organism (e.g. animals, plants, bacteria and viruses) and the artificial introduction of the genes to other completely different organisms (e.g. crop plants). The natural long-term evolution of species, which occurs after crossing similar organisms, has nothing to do with it. These new organisms acquire some new features, such as resistance to a particular herbicide. Genetic engineering typically uses viral genes for the insertion-promotion of foreign genes (i.e. genes resistant to antibiotics). The inserted genes are present in every cell of the plant.

Mutated organisms are artificial life forms that didn't exist in nature and, unlike traditional forms of biotechnology and plant production, eliminate the natural barriers that have been created between species through millions of years' worth of evolutionary process.

Thus, while crossing fish with a strawberry is impossible in nature, genetic engineering "succeeds" in doing it in the laboratory. Scientists extract a fish gene and implant it in a strawberry, thus creating an entirely new organism. Genetic engineering has the potential to use animal, plant, and even human genes.

Proponents of genetic engineering argue that mutated crops and resulting food products offer many advantages and can contribute effectively to the progress of humanity.

So, they promise to combat plant diseases and weeds with fewer drugs and pesticides leading to the protection of the environment, better production, higher agricultural incomes and combating hunger.

Why you should be against GMOs

My arguments are the same with those of Greenpeace, which I will mention, with the addition that, when humans (multinational companies), are motivated by wealth or fame and try to replace God by "creating" new organisms, then the results are catastrophic.

Greenpeace is against the release of GMOs, because the environmental dangers are inestimable and irreversible, the health effects on humans and animals are unknown, while the threat to biodiversity, ecological balance and food safety is immediate.

The deterioration of biodiversity, the increasing use of herbicides, weed and insect increased resistance to herbicides and insecticides, respectively, the gene transfer to other species (genetic pollution), and the release into the environment of organisms that may supplant natural related species, are among the risks that scientists have detected. If GMO are released into the environment, putting an end to the spread of their numbers would be impossible.

The health effects on humans and animals (through their feed) are unknown. The most probable dangers, as identified by physicians and geneticists are: emergence of new allergies, increasing resistance to antibiotics and toxic effects.

If people let government decide what foods they eat and what medicines they take, their bodies will soon be in as sorry a state as are the souls of those who live under tyranny [Thomas Jefferson (1743-1826) Third President of the United States].

SECTION 3: HERB THERAPY

Introduction-Advice

The use of herbs or herbal substances in treating diseases is as old as civilization itself. Surviving 5,000 year old written documents contain lists of plants, which were used in ancient China and Egypt. Hellenic mythology is full of references to medicinal herbs.

Humans aren't the only ones to use herbs. Chimpanzees eat an herb called aspilia, which is a paraciticidal and bactericidal. It has a bitter taste, as it becomes evident from their grimacing when eating it.

You should always remember that herbs should be treated as medicines. If you are taking other forms of medication, or if you are pregnant or possibly pregnant or have recently given birth or you are breastfeeding or if you have allergies, always consult your physician first before taking any herb.

Take note of the dosage and how often you use the herb. The herb dosage that I mention should be double-checked (by reading botany books and by applying the muscle test, p. 30). You shouldn't take them for more than four weeks. After you stop taking one kind of herb, switch to another, or stop all use for ten days and then continue taking the same herb.

In this book, the dosage mentioned is for adults. Children usually get half the adult dose, but consult your pediatrician first.

How to use and collect herbs

Herbs are used in the form of decoctions, infusions, compresses, poultices, tinctures, oils, essential oils, creams, ointments, juices, pills. You can use part of the plant or the entire plant.

Decoctions are made by boiling the hard parts of the plant (root, bark, or stems) in water (1 glass of water = 300 ml, 1 tea or water cup = 180 ml, 1 wineglass = 100 ml, 1 cup of Hellenic coffee = 60 ml).

Add a teaspoon of crushed herb in a small pan with water; boil it for ten minutes, and, after straining it, it's ready to drink. You can choose the temperature of the resulting beverage.

Infusions are prepared from the plant's soft parts, such as blossoms and leaves. Put a teaspoon of crushed herbs in a mug, along with boiling hot water, and leave it covered for twenty minutes. Stir it occasionally, strain it, and it's ready to drink.

In this book, every time there is a reference to a "decoction" or "infusion", it means a teaspoon of crushed herb (root, bark, or stem in decoction, blossoms and leaves in infusion) or mixture of herbs boiled in 300 ml water or added in 300 ml boiling hot water, to be taken half an hour before every meal, 3 times daily. Otherwise, the dosage or method of production and use will be mentioned.

Soak gauze or a piece of cotton in an infusion or a decoction and you have made a compress. In order to create a poultice, make a compress and place the boiled herbs inside of it. Compresses and poultices should be changed frequently (every two hours) and secured with cling film or an elastic bandage. The poultice should be quite hot, but in a temperature tolerable to the skin.

In order to prepare a tincture, the herb has to be soaked either in alcohol (rakee, vodka) or in apple vinegar and water for at least two weeks. Then, drain the liquid resulting from the blend, and you can drink it diluted in water or use it in a compress or ointment.

How to produce herbal oils and ointments: Put the herb (usually chopped) in a glass jar with olive oil (cold pressed or at least free of acids). Some other types of oil can also be used occasionally. You must leave it in a sunny or generally well-lit place for one or two months, but a lot less time could be needed, as it depends on the particular herb (e.g. a blend with garlic (allium sativum) is ready in two days). Strain the blend and you have made the oil (oil containing the fat soluble elements of the herb). If you don't have the luxury of waiting for one or two months, use a bain marie on low heat. Pour the olive oil with the crushed herbs in a small pot and place it in the bain marie, which you have filled with water. After two hours, remove the pot and strain the blend.

The most famous herb oil is St. John's wort oil (hypericum perforatum). You create it by mixing the crushed blossoms of the herb with olive oil and keeping the mixture in a sealed jar kept in the sun for a month; if you shake it well 4 times daily, it will be ready much sooner. The resulting blend is usually red. The chamomile (matricaria chamomilla) oil is made by using the herb's blossoms in a similar way.

You can use herb oils with beeswax (in a 4:1 volume ratio) to make an ointment. Boil the mixture above medium heat and, after the wax melts, pour it into jars. It will congeal after one or two minutes. It is advisable to sterilize the jars before use (i.e. by boiling them in water).

The garlic ointment is a very good antibiotic, just like ointments made with aromatic herbs [common thyme (thymus vulgaris), oregano (origanum vulgare), peppermint (mentha piperata), rosemary (rosmarinus officinalis), common sage (salvia officinalis), marjoram (origanum majorana), basil (ocimum basilicum), rock rose (cistus creticus), chamomile (matricaria chamomilla), etc.].

Anti-inflammatory ointments can be made by using: rock rose

(cistus creticus), St. John's wort [hypericum perforatum (balm)], ironwort (sideritis cretica), chamomile (matricaria chamomilla) or common marigold (calendula officinalis).

A face cream that can be used both as a day and a night cream (with anti-wrinkle action, revitalizing and invigorating) consists of: rock rose (cistus creticus), chamomile (matricaria chamomilla), wild mignonette (reseda lutea), Mediterranean cypress (cupressus sempervirens), rosemary (rosmarinus officinalis), common sage (salvia officinalis), St. John's wort (hypericum perforatum), common thyme (thymus vulgaris) and basil (ocimum basilicum).

As far as herbs are concerned, the way and time you collect and preserve them is of great importance. The farther they are from polluting sources (e.g. cities, factories, power cables, etc.) when collected, the better. It is best to collect them under the full moon, on a dry day, so the plant's juices are concentrated on its higher parts, the blossoms and the leaves. When you want to collect roots, usually in autumn, choose a moonless night. The collection of leaves should be done just before the full blossoming of the plants, and flowers should be gathered when fully open and just before they wither.

The gathered herbs should be dried in airy, dry places, with a temperature around 20-30°C, and should be used within the next eighteen months.

How to choose herbs

According to the Empedoclean-Hippocratic doctrine, humans and food are categorized in four types, depending on their temperature and moisture. They should use the appropriate herbs, according to their temperament.

The phlegmatic type needs warm and dry herbs: common thyme (thymus vulgaris), garlic (allium sativum), rosemary (rosmarinus officinalis), English lavender (lavandula officinalis), hyssop (hyssopus officinalis), ironwort (sideritis cretica), greater plantain (plantago major), fennel (foeniculum vulgare), common yarrow (achillea millefolium), coltsfoot (tussilago farfara), tansy (tanacetum vulgare), elderberry (sambucus nigra), basil (ocimum basilicum), motherwort (leonurus cardiac), micromeria juliana, greater celandine (chelidonium majus).

The melancholic type warm and moist herbs: Saint John's wort (hypericum perforatum), rock rose (cistus creticus), onion (allium cepa), cassia angustifolia, hellebore (helleborus cyclophyllus), common sage (salvia officinalis), marjoram (origanum majorana), common vervain (verbena officinalis), fenugreek (trigonella foenum-graecum), chickweed (stellaria media).

The choleric type needs cool and moist herbs: alpine skullcap (scutellaria alpina), chamomile (matricaria chamomilla), common lime (tilia europea), spearmint (mentha spicata), rhubarb, common dandelion (taraxacum officinalis), common chicory (cichorium intibus), heartsease (viola tricolor), dill (anethum graveolens), parsley (petroselinum sativum).

The sanguine type needs cool and dry herbs: common nettle (urtica dioica), lemon balm (melissa officinalis), figwort (scrophularia nodosa), greater burdock (arctium lappa), goosegrass (galium aparine), olive leaves (olea europea), barley (hordeum vulgare), peppermint (mentha piperata), pennyroal (mentha pulegium).

B. Chinese classify types of food and herbs depending on their taste which they see as their quintessence. Therefore, there are sweet, salty, spicy, sour and bitter herbs, and, of course, all of them, according to the Chinese worldview, are divided into yin and yang, two qualities that always coexist, but sometimes in different ratios. Illnesses are usually represented by a yang character, and the right thing would be to choose herbs of yin character, such as bitter [e.g. olive leaves (olea europea)] and sour ones [e.g. lemon balm (melissa officinalis)].

C. Paracelsus invented the theory of physiognomy, according to which a condition can be treated by administering herbs of the same nature as the organ and the patient's medical condition. You could apply, for example, St.John's wort (hypericum perforatum) balm to a wound (or drink it), because the herb's leaves appear to have wound-like holes, caused by its oils, and its oil is red like blood). In brain diseases, physicians recommend eating walnuts because the walnut possesses volutes and grooves, which look very similar to the brain's hemispheres. Carrots are a match to the eyes; beans to the kidneys; celery (apium graveolens) to the bones; eggplant, pears, avocado, and the leaves of alchemilla (alchemilla officinalis) to the womb and the cervix; sweet potato to the pancreas; olives to the ovaries; oranges to the chest; tomatoes to the heart; lungwort leaves (pulmonaria officinalis) to the lungs; figs to the testicles and sperm.

D. Hellenic people have a long tradition of folk medicine; grandmothers, grandfathers and monks have long devised either by experiments or by accident (during cases of human or animal diseases) or due to the insight of people of a high intellectual level, herbal recipes. These recipes are referred in the book as **grandma's remedies.**

E. Since you are already familiar with the muscle test for selecting food-substances, p. 30, you can apply it to yourself and discover which herb, which part of the plant (root, leaves, stem, fruit, blossoms, bark), what dosage, and what herb combinations suit you.

Herb Categories

Some of the herb categories, from which you can select herbs and undergo the muscle test for selecting food-substances, p. 30 are listed below:

Relaxants-anxiolytics-sedatives: chamomile (matricaria chamomilla), common lime (tilia europea), Saint John's wort (hypericum perforatum), lemon balm (melissa officinalis), marjoram (origanum majorana), spearmint (mentha spicata), pennyroyal (mentha pulegium), basil (ocimum basilicum), valerian (valeriana officinalis), purple passionflower (passiflora incarnate), English lavender (lavandula officinalis), common vervain (verbena officinalis), garden sage (salvia officinalis), common hop (humulus lupulus), alpine skullcap (scutellaria alpine), betony (stachys officinalis), olive tree (olea europea), saffron crocus (crocus sativus), laurel (laurus nobillis), rosemary (rosmarinus officinalis), common thyme (thymus vulgaris), lion's tail (leonurus cardiac), oat (avena sativa).

Anti-inflammatory: ironwort (sideritis cretica), Saint John's wort (hypericum perforatum), pot marigold (calendula officinalis), chamomile (matricaria chamomilla), rock rose (cistus creticus), white willow (salix alba), stinging nettle (urtica dioica), wild arum (arum maculatum), turmeric (curcuma longa), ginger, tansy (tanacetum vulgare), garden angelica (angelica archangelica), devil's claw (harpagophytum procumbens), oregano (origanum vulgare), common thyme (thymus vulgaris), common lime (tilia europea), fenugreek (trigonella foenum graecum), great mullein (verbascum thapsus), garlic (allium sativum), onion (allium cepa), mugwort (artemisia vulgaris), coltsfoot (tussilago farfara), marsh mallow (althea officinalis), menyanthes (menyanthes trifoliate), olive tree (olea europea), yarrow (achillea millefolium), greater plantain (plantago major), arnica (arnica montana), eastern teaberry (gaultheria procumbens), aleppo pine (pinus halepensis), potato, elderberry (sambucus nigra).

Bactericidal-fungicidal-antiviral-paraciticidal: garlic (allium sativum), common thyme (thymus vulgaris), rosemary (rosmarinus officinalis), oregano (origanum vulgare), laurel (laurus nobillis), savory (satureja thymbra), common sage (salvia officinalis), Saint John's wort (hypericum perforatum), lemon balm (melissa officinalis), elderberry (sambucus nigra), great mullein (verbascum thapsus), rock rose (cistus creticus), chamomile (matricaria chamomilla), English lavender (lavandula officinalis), cinnamon (cinnamomum zeylanicum), milkvetch (astragalus spruneri), basil (ocimum basilicum), ironwort (sideritis cretica), onion (allium cepa), olive tree (olea europea), rue (ruta graveolens), pot marigold (calendula officinalis), fennel (foeniculum vulgare), milk thistle (silybum marianum), common witch hazel, (hamamelis virginiana), hyssop (hyssopus officinalis), echinacea (echinacea angustifolia), common bistort (polygonum bistarta), barley (hordeum vulgare), upright pellitory (parietaria diffusa), arbutus tree (arbutus officinalis), common yarrow (achillea millefolium), common bearberry (arctostaphylos uva ursi), narrow-leaved paperbark (melaleuca alternifolia), manna ash (fraxinus ornus), mugwort (artemisia vulgaris), Cretan ditanny (origanum dictamnus).

Pharmaceutical companies are trying to analyze herbs and isolate the miracle ingredient that will cure or combat a disease. When they find the ingredient, they decide whether it is cheaper and feasible to synthesize it in their laboratories or if it will cost less to create plantations of the particular herb. Nowadays, twenty five per cent of medication available is derived from plants, which have been analyzed by pharmaceutical companies.

In Chronic Obstructive Pulmonary Disease (dyspnea, cough, sputums), also known as Smoker's Disease, which appeared in Europe after Jean Nicot introduced tobacco plants in Europe during the 16th century, physicians prescribe tiotropium bromide (under the trade name spiriva). The pharmaceutical industry uses the extract of the plant corkwood (duboisa mycoporoides), which is systematically cultivated in Brazil, in order to produce it. This medication was a small revolution in the treatment of COPD, because it was the first inhaled anticholinergic to be taken one time a day with a very good bronchodilator effect that led to an obvious improvement of the respiratory parameters.

Bromhexine and ambroxol are the active substances of the expectorants bisolvon and mucosolvan respectively, and derive from the plant malabar nut (justicia adhatoda), which is cultivated in Pakistan.

The bulb of the plant narcissus is systematically cultivated in Belgium, because it's the source of the substance galantamine, which is the active ingredient of revinyl, a medicine used for treating Alzheimer's disease.

The famous fava beans contain the well-known amino acid L-Dopa, which is the main drug used against Parkinson's disease. In particular, 250g of fava beans amount to 125mg L-Dopa/12,5mg Carvidopa.

Acetyl salicylic acid, sold under the trade name aspirin, can be found in the form of its precursor (salicylic acid) in the cortex of the white willow tree (salix alba), from which it was discovered. Since then, chemical laboratories synthesize it from its basic elements.

The difference between the herb and the medicine is that an herb doesn't have just a single miraculous ingredient, but a variety of them, which aid or antagonize each other, so that people can be the recipients of their therapeutic effect.

"Panacea herbs"

Only God cures everything but "Panacea herbs" means that the following herbs will probably cure everything.

There are 7,000 species of plants in Hellas. In the following web pages, you will find many detailed photos of eight of the most common herbs found in Hellas, under their Latin names, and their descriptions, so that you learn how to identify them (plants have different names in many parts of Hellas, something which makes their identification impossible).

http://flowersofymittos.blogspot.gr/
http://floraattica.blogspot.gr/
http://rosa-sempervirens.blogspot.gr/
http://floraolympus.blogspot.gr/
http://florakristonia.blogspot.gr/
http://eliastselos.blogspot.gr/
http://greekflora.gr/
http://plant171.blogspot.gr/
http://floraofsyros.blogspot.gr/
http://hellenicnature.blogspot.gr/
http://melissokomikonergastirion.blogspot.gr
http://floracytherea.blogspot.gr
http://floraamorgina.blogspot.gr/
http://luirig.altervista.org/flora/taxa/floraindice.php (This web page is about the Italian flora, which is similar to Hellenic, and you can also find many detailed pictures there).

Apart from the characteristic indications mentioned under each herb, the muscle test for selecting food-substances, p. 30 would be of great assistance. You only have to mention the herb's name and then ascertain if your hand is getting stronger, and then repeat it in order to see how many times you should drink tea brewed from this herb. Be careful, as the following "panacea herbs" are not recommended for pregnant women.

Rock rose (cistus creticus)

The rock rose is the plant with the highest content of polyphenols in Europe, thus capable of destroying free radicals, and has a high antioxidant activity.

Studies from German universities showed that it protects the heart four times better than red wine and that it is twenty times more antioxidant than fresh lemon juice. The rock rose detoxifies the body and eliminates toxic heavy metals generated by cigarette smoke, dental fillings and environmental pollution.

It is an herb with anti-wrinkle and anti-aging action, and excellent for skins with acne and neurodermatitis.

A potent anti-inflammatory, it is also very useful in treating lumbago, sciatica, tendonitis and autoimmune diseases (lupus erythematosus, rheumatoid arthritis, etc.).

Rock rose's anti-haemorrhagic qualities make it useful in treating menorrhagia and nose bleeds (by inserting a rock rose solution soaked cotton ball in the nostril).

A natural relaxant, it is suitable for treating anxiety, insomnia and chronic fatigue syndrome. Likewise, it is very good in the treatment of gastritis and colitis.

Since it is antimicrobial, antiviral and antifungal, studies have shown that it acts against staphylococous aureus, escherichia coli, candida albicans and helicobacter pylori.

In combination with its diuretic action, this herb is useful against urinary tract infections and prostatitis. Rock rose blossoms are suitable for treating kidney stones. It has been used against obesity and some forms of tumors since antiquity.

Dosage: one teaspoon of dried or fresh grated leaves in a teacup, four times a day. Boil them for two minutes.

The small petioles (stems), where leaves, blossoms and flower buds grow are also of medicinal value.

So far, there haven't been any known side-effects.

Olive tree (Olea europea)

The leaves of the olive tree have the following properties: they are antiseptic, antimicrobial, antifungal, antiviral, antihypertensive, diuretic; they protect the heart (by dilating the coronary vessels); they alleviate cardiac arrhythmias, psoriasis and toothache; they lower cholesterol, blood sugar, and curb one's appetite; they are astringent (useful when dealing with diarrhea and hemorrhoids), antipyretic, antioxidant (so, useful to cancer patients), alleviate rheumatisms-arthritis, and helpful in either relaxing or energizing your body or mind.

The olive tree's bark, which is collected during spring from the tree's young branches, lowers blood sugar levels and acts as an antipyretic.

Virgin olive oil (which is produced by simply pressing the olives without heating the resulting pulp or adding any chemicals) is part of the famous Mediterranean diet and is the elixir of youth and longevity. It can be used to aid constipation or gastric hypersecretion; it can also combat dry skin, dry hair and dandruff; it can be used as a massage oil plain or with other herbs, as a diluter or natural additive (booster) in herb extracts or medication and it can also be applied on wounds, plain or mixed with red wine.

For not easily treatable skin ulcers-sores (of diabetics, for example), you can prepare an ointment by mixing 1 tsp. of sweet virgin olive oil, 1 tsp. pure honey and 500mg penicillin powder. Apply it three times a day on the wound.

Olive trees growing in the mountains and anywhere far away from pollution and pesticides are generally more preferable.

Here are some instructions on how to prepare an olive leave decoction: Boil ten dry, intact and free of pesticide, olive leaves in two cups of water for 15 minutes at 80° C. Drink half of it in the morning and the other half in the evening (keep the blend in a tightly sealed jar in the refrigerator). You should consult your physician for the dosage and when to take it, especially if it is to be taken by children.

Dr D. Lambropoulos recommends the following recipe for serious medical conditions: Put a glass of olive leaves (110g) and two glasses of water (bottled, preferably non-chlorinated) in a blender, at a ratio of 1:2. In the beginning, just add a small amount of water. Then, work the blender for three minutes, while gradually adding the remaining water. You should stop the blender every half a minute or so, in order to make sure that the mixture doesn't get too much heated. According to Dr. Lambropoulos' advice, you must drink 100 ml of the extract, three times a day (i.e. morning, afternoon and evening), before or after a meal, for at least four months. To offset the bitter taste, you can add some fruit juice or a little honey.

The therapeutic range of olive leaves (olea europea) is large (more than 5,000), indicating that olive leaves are safe herbs.

Garlic (allium sativum)

Garlic is self-sown and can be found all over Hellas during spring and summer. Being able to recognize it will be very useful because garlic is a profoundly beneficial food.

Modern studies confirm the following benefits:

Lower arterial blood pressure and levels of total cholesterol. Prevention of arterial thrombosis, and the development of atheromatous plaque. Lower cardiovascular risk markers in smokers and obese individuals.

Eradication of Helicobacter pylori, germs, viruses, fungi and intestinal parasites.

Beneficial results against a multitude of diseases, such as cancer, diabetes, Alzheimer, influenza, acne, genital warts, herpes, osteoarthritis, urinary tract infection, immune and cardiovasculatory disorders; also, improved sexual drive.

An ancient anti-rheumatic recipe is the topical (joint) application of a poultice made from ten crushed garlic cloves mixed in a litre of vinegar for at least ten days.

Epidemiological studies have shown that there is an inverse relationship between garlic consumption and the death rate of many types of cancer, such as: prostate cancer, lung cancer, endometrial cancer, skin cancer, gastrointestinal tract cancer, liver cancer, breast cancer and blood malignancies.

It is helpful in the recovery from alcohol, smoking and drug addiction.

Patients who take anticoagulant medication must show caution when consuming garlic, as it displays antithrombotic properties.

Dosage: The suggested adult dose is generally four grams (up to three cloves) of garlic a day or a tablet of garlic (300mg) two or three times a day.

An old recipe:

325g peeled garlic clones

200g pure alcohol (ethanol) 95%

50ml of water or milk

Crush the garlic with a porcelain, glass, or wooden pestle (don't use a mixer, because it mustn't come in contact with metal objects) and put it in a jar with the alcohol. Mix them together and store it in the fridge for eleven days, shaking it well daily. On the eleventh day, strain the mixture and store the resulting solution back in the fridge. You can preserve the thick residue in olive oil and keep it in the fridge for even up to three years (during this process, don't forget to wear latex gloves). You can use the olive oil strained from the residue to treat stubborn open wounds.

Add a few drops of the solution in 50ml of water or milk and after ten minutes (to allow the alcohol to evaporate) you may drink it. It is to be taken thirty minutes before meals.

The following table shows how many drops to add:

Days	Morning	Afternoon	Evening
1st	1 drop	2 drops	3 drops
2nd	4	5	6
3rd	7	8	9
4th	10	11	12
5th	13	14	15
6th	15	14	13
7th	12	11	10
8th	9	8	7
9th	6	5	4
10th	3	2	1
11th	25	25	25
12th	25	25	25

The dosage is larger for cancer patients. The garlic needed is 525g and the alcohol 300g. You can start with 40 drops in 60ml of water or milk for the first ten days (in cases of metastasis add 50 drops in 70ml) and then continue with 25 drops, until you have taken all of the solution (always 3 times daily).

The solution is sufficient for persons with body weights between 30 to 110 kg. As a precaution, the above treatment should not be resumed no sooner than after five years.

Garlic also has some other unusual uses. It can act as insect repellent, pesticide, and its juice can be used to make glue.

Summer asphodel (asphodelus aestivus)

The summer asphodel has been used since antiquity, especially in times of famine: its tubers, which contain starch, are edible and they can be used to produce sticky flour, which is called "aspho-delion". Tubers are very nutritious because of the large amount of starch and glue they contain.

Medically speaking, the most useful parts of the roots are their yellow cylindrical tubers. Autumn is the best season for their collection.

The summer asphodel is very effective against asthmatic bronchitis, if given as a decoction, and for healing wounds and chilblains in poultice form. It is also known for its expectorant, cardiotonic, diuretic, spasmolytic, emetic and antibiotic action. Finally, it is very interesting that, if combined with wine, the resulting blend makes a very impressive tonic.

Hippocrates, Dioscorides and Pliny, said that the roots were cooked in ashes and then eaten. There is a quite popular Turkish dish called Çirişotu, which is made with the plant's cooked leaves.

In traditional folk medicine, stems and tubers are used to treat hemorrhoids, nephritis and wounds. The Palestinian people's folk medicine still uses the summer asphodels to heal bumps growing between the joints of the hands or feet.

The roots of the plant, if dried and boiled in water, produce a sticky substance that is mixed with cereals or potatoes in some countries, in order to make asphodel bread.

In Spain, and some other countries, the roots are used as animal feed, especially for sheep. They are also a real delicacy to wild hogs.

During some difficult times in Hellenic history (i.e. during times of war or poverty), people collected asphodel tubers and shoots, boiled them and used them for sustenance.

When its powder is mixed with cold water, it swells and becomes strong adhesive glue.

Common or stinging nettle (urtica dioica)

It's another "panacea plant", but also edible (its shoots can be eaten raw and the rest of the plant can be eaten boiled). All of its parts are useful (leaves, stems, seeds, blossoms and roots).

It's anti-inflammatory, anti-rheumatic (useful in sciatica, auto-immune diseases and arthritis), anti-anaemic, blood-producing, blood-purifying, suitable for those suffering from eczema-derma-titis due to poor diet, astringent (i.e. suitable for diarrhea, hem-orrhoids, gastritis with gastric hypersecretion) anti-haemorrhagic (increases blood clotting, suitable for nosebleeds, excessive men-ses, haemoptysis), diuretic (very useful in hematuria and gout), antidiabetic, lithoclastic (in Epirus of Hellas, they drink a glass of decoction of a teaspoon of crushed seeds every morning), anti-allergic, useful in liver and bile disorders and against constipation (by eating boiled, crushed seeds), expectorant, useful in disorders of the spleen, combats hair loss and dandruff, it gives hair a spe-cial shine (drink an infusion and rinse your hair with a decoction or tincture of the herb's leaves and root), sedative and milk-pro-ducing in nursing mothers. It has also been reported that it helps in children's development, if mixed with carrot juice at a ratio 1:3, and that it is anticarcinomatous. Foot baths with stinging nettle (urtica dioica) decoction help in dealing with the reduced circula-tion of the lower limbs (ulcers, gangrene), wounds and eczema.

Dosage: a tablespoon of crushed stinging nettle (urtica dioica) added in 200g of water, one to three times a day.

It should be avoided by elderly people prone to thrombosis and by women with uterine fibroids.

Oregano (origanum vulgare)

The antibiotic properties of oregano have been recognized in recent times and, though the plant is self-sown, it is cultivated in large areas; the extracted oregano essence is used as an animal antibiotic.

Certain animals, instinctively knowing its antibiotic, hemostatic, analgesic and healing action, apply it to their wounds.

It particularly helps with diarrhea, respiratory infections, constipation, intestinal peristalsis, hiccups, belching, flatulence (abdominal bloating), digestion (i.e. it increases the secretion of gastric acid and thus helps combat gastritis caused by diminished secretion of gastric fluids) and anorexia.

It can be used against anaemia, as a sedative, antispasmodic, diaphoretic, antirheumatic and anticonvulsant; it is useful when dealing with asthma, whooping cough, spasmodic cough and painful menstruation (dysmenorrhea).

It is recommended to be drank as an infusion (mix one teaspoon of the herb in half a glass of boiled water and leave it to brew for half an hour), taken one to three times a day.

St. John's wort (hypericum perforatum)

St. John's wort (hypericum perforatum) is one of the thirty-five hypericum species that can be found in Hellas. It is another "herb panacea", which is also called valsamohorto, valsamo (in Mt Athos and Arcadia), spathohorto (Epirus), ayoudhouras (Crete), the Prodromos' herb, valsamaki, balsam, leichinohorto, kapetouri (Messinia), pseirovotano, helonovorto (Cephalonia), koktsoudhi, periki, kopsovotano, ghouthoura, staritha, spathidha.

Your hand will be stained red if you rub it between your fingers. Hypericin and hyperforin are the main and most studied chemical substances found in hypericum perforatum.

It is used to treat mild-moderate depression; in 1988, its total sales reached the six billion US dollars in Europe. It is preferred because it lacks the main side effect of many antidepressants (i.e. sexual dysfunction). The plant is also an immune system stimulant, antibiotic, antimicrobic (used in respiratory and urinary tract infections, gastroenteritis, vaginitis, dermatitis), antifungal, anthelminthic, antiviral (it is even given to AIDS patients) and antipyretic. Its healing, antihaemorrhoidal and anti-inflammatory properties make it very useful in treating burns, gastritis, colitis, tendonitis, arthritis, fibromyalgia and back pain.

Its antineuralgic action is also beneficial in treating lumbar sciatica, prosopalgia, shingles; its diuretic action is used in treating prostatitis and prostatic hypertrophy; its anticarcinomatous action is used in cases of leukemia, brain glioblastoma and bladder cancer. It is also antiepileptic, antihaemorrhagic, anticteric, detoxifying, antioxidant; it protects the bone marrow from radiation; it is emmenagogic, relaxant and a mild sedative; useful in treating headaches, insomnia, faintness, anorexia; beneficial in treating eczema and leg ulcers; and it is also very good for people who wish to quit drinking alcohol or smoking. It was called spathohorto (i.e. shordwort) because it used to be applied on sword wounds.

Dosage: infusion of hypericum perforatum blossoms, up to 3 times daily or one pill of 300mg hypericin, up to 3 times daily. The herb's oil, (which is prepared by creating a mixture of its blossoms and oil, placing it in a tightly sealed glass jar, and leaving it in the sun for 40 days), is usually red and used for topical applications in cases of myalgia, neuralgia, tendonitis, dermatitis, burns, bedsores and wounds.

Side effects-interactions with medication: Hypericin may very rarely cause a photosensitivity reaction-photosensitization to people with light skin, so it is recommended to avoid prolonged exposure to sunlight after taking hypericum perforatum.

If you take antidepressants, contraceptives, anticoagulants, cardiotonics, immunosuppressants, anti-asthmatics, antivirals, opioids, chemoprophylactics, or other medication, your primary physician must be informed.

Wild arum (arum maculatum, dracunculus vulgaris)

It belongs to the Araceae family comprising approximately of 750 species. It should be noted that the fruit, leaves, stem and root of the plant are all poisonous.

The main toxin it contains is called aroine, which is unstable and can be neutralized by properly drying or cooking the herb. Aroine is a skin irritant, and toxic to the central nervous system. That's why you need to use gloves when handling the herb.

The roots are usually harvested in the spring or autumn. They are tuberous roots (just like in potatoes), and have medicinal properties. They act as antirheumatics, antiasthmatics, antitussives, anti-pertussis, expectorants, anti-defluxion, anti-tuberculosis, antihaemorrhagic, antihaemorrhoidal and anti-diarrheal.

Its fruit extract destroys nasal polyps (be careful of its caustic-toxic action). It is also used as a poultice in order to treat arthritis and orchitis. Dioscorides, the most famous pharmacologist and botanist of Classical antiquity, mentions that it heals gastritis, ulcers, and that it is an aphrodisiac.

I have also heard of cases where it has been used as an anti-carcinomatous medication (with great success, in some cases) and it is particularly effective against cancers of the gastrointestinal tract.

Dosage-preparation: Wear gloves, start peeling the roots (exactly like you do with potatoes), and then dry them, or crush them into a mortar, until they turn into a fine powder, or grate them (as you would do with cheese).

If you grate the roots, you get a white, slightly moist, mush. Mix the mush with a little flour (any type will do), then shape the mixture into small balls, the size of small chickpeas.

You can create about 100 balls from a dracunculus vulgaris tuberous root. Then, they should be kept in the freezer. You can eat the first ball the next day, giving the root time to lose its toxicity. Wait for the ball to thaw for ten minutes (to make it easier to swallow) and then swallow it without chewing it first; because it will leave a burning feeling in your mouth (some combine it with a bit of honey).

Eat one such ball or drink one cups of tea made from the crushed arum maculatum, 3 times daily.

SECTION 4: HYDROTHERAPY

Thermal baths

In 850 BC, Homer writes that Odysseus, when he and his men ended up in Circe's palace, was offered the use of the bathing rooms, as an honor from his host, and then he was showered with expensive perfumes.

Hydrotherapy flourished in ancient Hellas, in Hippocrates' time (i.e. 460-370 BC). In fact, the Asclepia, which were healing sanctuaries, were built next to thermal springs.

Thermal baths were very popular among the Romans, who used eighty springs for therapeutic purposes.

After the 6th century BC, the Byzantine Empire strict Christian morality came in direct contrast to the loose sexual morals and orgies, which occurred in thermal bath towns.

In Western Europe, during the Middle Ages, there was a strong polemic against hydrotherapy. But, during the 17th and 18th century, the study of thermal springs' chemical analysis led to the revival of thermal bath towns.

In 1830, J. Kapodistrias, governor of Hellas, sent medical doctors to the island of Kythnos, in order to study the local springs. During the reign of King Othon, the first hydrotherapy centre in modern Hellas was created on the same island.

In 1938, the Department of Clinical Hydrotherapy and Medical

Climatology was founded in the Medical School of the University of Athens, but it was abolished in 1955, due to the lack of interest shown by physicians and by the State for the study of thermal waters.

Pharmaceutical and surgical medicine prevailed entirely; today, the ancient and timelessly proven therapeutic method of hydrotherapy is considered to be a complementary and alternative form of medicine.

In modern Hellas, thermal baths are correlated to seniors citizens. Thermal baths towns become some kind of retirement communities every year between August and September.

In many foreign countries, thermal baths and spas are associated with enjoyment and relaxing weekends. They are mostly preferred by young people. Thermal waters are used to fill modern swimming pools, which are equipped with special water jets for fun and therapeutic purposes (whirlpool baths). European countries with cold climate have created open air swimming pools, which communicate with enclosed heated spaces, so that their citizens can swim in warm thermal waters, even in open swimming pools, all year round.

In European areas with thermal springs, the waters are shared between all surrounding hotels, and spa tourism is going through a new golden era.

There are 752 thermal springs scattered all over Hellas. Older people, despite the intractable diseases, keep visiting them as they realize the benefits to their health. Young people, who have started having various health problems from an early age, should take advantage of what Hellenic nature offers.

The relaxation that thermal waters offer is ideal for young people suffering from anxiety issues concerning their professional advancement and romantic relationships.

Lately, Hellenic people living near thermal springs have come to realize that its waters are not just for the elderly. The fact that certain illnesses have started affecting people from an earlier age, and younger people's tendency to avoid medication and surgery, have contributed to this change in opinion.

I often visit the thermal waters of Eastern Continental Hellas and I have seen many children playing in the warm shallow waters, something which fills me with joy. Some families with young children even go for picnics near thermal springs.

You shouldn't think that these springs are unsuitable for you due to all the elderly people using them, because their waters are constantly being renewed by small streams snaking out from smaller or larger openings in the ground, while larger rivulets of the previous used waters stream out of the thermal pools or ponds. No fish or plants can survive in thermal waters due to their temperature and composition; you can safely enjoy your swim there.

Organized spas, which capitalize on the waters of thermal springs, have individual bathtubs where it's mandatory that you shower first before having a soak. The thermal water in these bathtubs isn't stationary either, as there is continuous water flow.

The words "thermal waters" and "spas" have been mentioned many times in this section, but it should also be noted that in Hellas they are called "healing waters", because there is a traditional belief that they can heal diseases. This belief exists thanks to people who regained their health after taking thermal baths, or animals which were healed after accidentally soaking in a thermal spring. Scientists have discovered that thermal waters contain minerals.

The waters of a spring are called mineral when they contain an increased concentration of solid or gaseous components, or when they are of a high temperature, or when they contain a small concentration of a component with known therapeutic effects (i.e. hydrogen sulfide, radium emissions, iron, lithium, iodine, etc.).

Thermal-mineral waters contain dissolved solids in quantities greater than 1 g per every kg of water.

These waters are found in great depths due to tectonic faults (submerging of Aegis) or due to volcanic eruptions. The high temperatures that are prevalent in these depths push them towards the surface. Trace elements (iron, sulfur, magnesium, radium, sodium, chlorine, bromine, iodine etc.) and gases (carbon dioxide, oxygen, hydrogen, hydrogen sulfide, etc.) trail along their side on their way to the surface.

The waters of thermal springs are characterized according to their mineral component with the highest concentration (e.g.: sulfides, chlorinated, radioactive, high-iron, bromide and iodide). At the same time, the waters have a certain degree of acidity (acidic, neutral and alkaline), and that's why they are described accordingly (e.g.: alkaline sulfide thermal spring, such as those in the Hellenic villages New Apollonia and Smokovo).

There are 229 thermal springs on the Hellenic islands, 156 in Central Hellas, 114 in the Peloponnese, 115 in Macedonia, 57 in Thessaly, 25 in Thrace and 77 of them are officially recognized as thermo-mineral springs. The ones largely or frequently used are 348.

Each one has its own characteristics (composition, temperature) and completely different effects on each patient. There might be some generalizations about the therapeutic action of particular thermal springs, but one has to try a certain spring in order to determine whether it's partially or completely right for them.

The effectiveness of thermal waters lies in their temperature and their chemical composition. They stimulate the cutaneous nerve endings and have a great effect on the human body through the absorption of trace elements from the skin and respiratory system.

There are many excellent thermal springs in Central Hellas, and one of the best is located in a small village called Damasta (10 km from Lamia, near Thermopylae), a spring that anyone can visit free of charge throughout the year. It is open around the clock, and is always lighted, thanks to the initiative of the district mayors. It belongs to the Hellenic State but the will of the land-owner, who bequeathed it to them, states that it should always be open to all people and that no one is to make any profit out of it. This thermal spring is a natural small paradise that God so generously offered to his unworthy children.

The thermal waters of Damasta (three springs which form a pond and two pools with a small difference in temperature) are also called Psoroneria (i.e. Psoriasis waters), but that does not mean that all the people suffering from psoriasis will benefit from bathing in these springs. It might be possible that another one could be a better match for a particular patient. These waters are also known for their cosmetic properties. If you are subjected to a full thermal bath treatment (twenty-one baths in at least fifteen days) and you see no improvement, look for another thermal spring, and consider other treatment options.

The pond measures one metre in depth, about 15 metres in width, and about 100 meters in length. In some parts of the pond, it feels like you are taking a bath in soda water, because of the hydrogen sulfide gas emitted from multiple small holes in the bed of the pond before making its way to the surface. The springs have a rotten egg smell (because of the hydrogen sulphide they contain) but, surprisingly, after five minutes of soaking in the water, the smell is no longer an issue.

Sulfur is present in large quantities in the skin, articular cartilage and the thyroid as a trace element. It has been proven that the sulfur contained in thermal water penetrates the skin and reaches the joints. A past remedy involved treating skin diseases by placing suplhur on the affected person's skin.

Some also use the mud that can be found next to the springs for mud baths.

It is also very important that in 2007 they placed a special ramp in the pond for the easier access of people with disabilities.

Avoid visit the springs between August and early September,

because they are filled with people from dawn until late in the evening. You will constantly see people arriving in private coaches, local buses and private cars.

If you visit during the summer, be ready to be besieged by mosquitoes after dusk. The thermal springs of Damasta are open air springs, after all.

The thermal waters in the city of Kamena Vourla, being radioactive and chlorinated, are considered to be especially beneficial in rheumatic and arthritic diseases, neuralgia, paresis (motion impairment) and in atherosclerosis. It was also what healed my three-year-old daughter's atopic dermatitis (eczema). The treatment lasted for three days and it involved swimming six times in Galini hotel's pool.

The irony is that I had been told that these waters were radioactive and not suitable for minors. When I asked them for scientific proof to back their claims, they remained silent (I knew there wasn't any).

My daughter was finally allowed entrance, due to my medical status and because I assumed all responsibility, and since then, these thermal springs have become a favorite holiday and preventative medicine destination for my family and I.

You shouldn't feel apprehensive over using the radioactive waters of these famous and much-frequented thermal springs, because the radium they contain is in gas form and not in the dangerous form of salts. If the space is properly ventilated, then there will be no problem. The same patients have been visiting them for decades and they always leave them feeling refreshed.

If there was Chernobyl-like radiation, wouldn't the swimmers, or people working at the springs have had displayed certain symptoms? Moreover, scientists have measured the levels of radioactivity in famous thermal springs and none of them recommended that they should be avoided.

Do not hesitate to do things people have been doing for

centuries without any side effects. Try out things, take initiatives and form your own opinion.

The thermal waters of Thermopylae are listed as beneficial to asthma and lung diseases (taking deep breaths while being immersed neck-deep in the water is a form of treatment), but I know that most of the local population (esp. Lamia's citizens) visit them to treat the symptoms of spinal disorders.

Whenever I visit, I see caravans with foreign plates parked next to the thermal springs and foreigners enjoying the waters.

The high temperature of these waters (i.e.: 40°C) makes them ideal for winter swimming at any time of the day, and no matter how low the atmospheric temperature might be.

In the thermal spring of Ypati (Central Hellas), the brochure of the Tourism Development Company, which manages the spring, mentions the following therapeutic indications:

Diseases and vascular syndromes

Arterial hypertension, deficiency of the heart's coronary arteries, endarteritis of the lower limbs (intermittent claudication), phlebitis

Heart diseases, diseases of the heart valves, minor heart failures.

Disorders of the heart and the nervous system, tachycardia, arrhythmias.

Skin diseases, eczema, dermatitis and other skin issues.

Disorders of peripheral nerves and muscles, paralysis, muscle atrophy.

Arthritis in many of its forms.

It is a fact that the thermal spring of Ypati has a temperature of 33°C and it is quite rich in carbonic acid, hydrogen sulfide, chlorine and sodium; a unique thermal spring, world-famous for its chemical composition.

Dr. Fokas, the Professor of Hydrology at the Athens University has provided the characteristics of the thermal spring of Palaiovrachas (Central Hellas) listed on a public notice posted in one of the spring' surrounding buildings: temperature 26.5°C, radioactivity 0.40, very faint smell of hydrogen sulphide, hydrogen index 9.6, metaboric acid 0.0201, unsuitable for drinking. Therapeutic indications: arthritis, diabetes, psoriasis, kidney stones, gall stones, cholecystitis, hepatitis, asthma, chronic bronchitis, chronic enterocolitis, light dermatopathies.

When you step into the waters, you will find many people already there. The half an hour soak people usually have, passes more quickly by having discussions with the other swimmers. You will hear many of their experiences, many stories and many opinions regarding the healing properties of thermal waters.

My recommendation is to stay in the water for as long as you feel comfortable and relaxed, without counting the time you spend in the spring. If you begin to feel tired, bored or any kind of discomfort, you should get out of the water. The time spent in hot springs is considerably less than the time spent in thermal springs, because the latter's temperature is closer to your body's temperature.

Many people ask me if they can combine thermal baths with swimming in the sea. You may fearlessly combine these two different types of swimming, but only go for a swim at the sea some time later than your thermal spring soak, and only after the pores of your skin, which opened after soaking in the warm thermal waters, close. The older you are, the more time you will need before swimming in the sea. Three hours are required on average.

Swimming in the sea is more beneficial to those who like the cold and moisture, (i.e. relatively healthy choleric types). The more melancholic or the more phlegmatic someone is, the more they want warmer, and with a higher salt content, sea waters. But, don't forget that during summertime even the last two types might feel exhausted from the heat, and seek cool, moist places. Winter swimmers enjoy their swimming sessions because they provide them with cold and moistness. This is an indication that they have a hot and dry disposition, which means they are choleric.

Patients suffering from heart disease, or venous insufficiency of the lower limps, should avoid hot waters. They should prefer lukewarm waters (e.g.: thermal spring of Ypati). Women who are menstruating should stay away from thermal baths, and pregnant women should avoid hot waters. All swimmers should be careful after soaking in a thermal spring. They should dry themselves immediately and thoroughly, in case they find themselves in a sudden gust of wind while their skin pores are still open. Elderly people should avoid taking thermal baths on windy days. Young people shouldn't drive their motorcycles if they have not dried themselves well, or don't have the proper protective gear.

You should have no worries about taking your children with you to thermal springs. Just keep in mind to let them spend just a little time in hot waters and advise them not to get in and out very often, especially when it is windy.

I strongly advise you to visit a thermal spring during your family holidays. The best season for such a visit is the warm days of spring and the first half of summer. Visit and get to know as many thermal springs as possible.

Finally, let me give you a recipe for creating your own thermal bath at home (God has provided you with everything you might need): Add as much natural sea salt as you wish in your bathtub, or in a basin, filled with hot or lukewarm water (salt dissolves more easily in hot water). Then, you can add large quantities of already boiled herbs (i.e. herbs which are beneficial to your condition, or help you relax, e.g. pinus halepensis).

People who gain many benefits from thermal baths (at a temperature of 37°C) are the ones who need warmth and moisture, which means they are melancholic types, with a cool and dry disposition.

Mud therapy, mud baths

Several swimmers, after they finish with their bath, take mud found in specific points adjacent to the thermal springs or from the bed of the spring and proceed to smear mud on certain areas of their body because they feel pain or suffer from skin disease or feel quite stiff. They wait for the mud to dry under the strong sun and then they start feeling the dried mud pulling at their skin, and giving relief to that particular area of their body. The dried mud should be left on the body for half an hour and then rinsed off with warm thermal water.

Avoid taking a mud bath when a strong wind is blowing, because the skin pores open with the mud bath and the harmful effects of the wind will affect your body. Also take care not to smear mud or take a mud bath when you have open wounds on your body, because there is the possibility of getting a skin infection.

There are some thermal springs, such as the ones in the city of Philippi in Kavala, where people bathe in mud pits. In fact, these thermal springs have a special crane, which is used for lowering disabled patients into the mud pits.

Phlegmatic types, being of a cold and moist disposition, benefit greatly from mud therapy, since they crave warmth and dryness.

Water (drinking) therapy

This therapy is used to treat disorders of the gastrointestinal and urinary tract, and of the skin; also others, such as dyspeptic syndrome, constipation, urinary tract infection, gallstones, biliary stasis, psoriasis and eczema.

Salts, small stones and waste products are swept away and

expelled from the body as the water passes through the intestinal, biliary and urinary pathways. The drinking therapy should be done in the morning while you are unfed or many hours after having (light) meals and with extra care from those who have prostate problems, active peptic ulcers and severe liver diseases.

There are many famous Hellenic drinking water springs, such as: the Korpi spring in the town of Vonitsa in Aitoloakarnania, the Xynou Nerou spring in the city of Florina, the water springs in the town of Platystomo in Fthiotida and springs of Loutraki in Cornithia.

Inhalation therapy

The thermal springs you can use when following this therapy are the ones in Smokovo, Kyllini, Thermopylae, Caiaphas and Amarantou (in the prefecture of Ioannina, 40 Km from the town of Konitsa).

Their waters are sulphide, except of those of Amarantou, whose waters are calcic and suitable for treating chronic respiratory diseases, such as asthma, chronic bronchitis, chronic rhinitis, chronic pharyngitis and chronic laryngitis.

Steam baths

The steam bath can be for the whole body (sauna) or for a particular affected area of the body. The steam causes sweating, resulting in the expelling of secretions (detoxification). Many patients (particularly those with cold extremities) need the heat which seeps into the body.

People with cardiac disorders and respiratory problems are advised against using a sauna.

If you suffer from lower back pain, then the topical application of a steam bath could be the primary (inexpensive, relatively simple and, most importantly, effective) solution. Lie face down and naked on top of a bed, which is covered with a towel. Carefully place a pan of boiling hot steaming water (just removed from the hob) between your knees and cover your waist and legs (but not your back) with a linen blanket.

Be careful not to touch the pot or spill hot water on yourself because you may suffer burns (get one or two friends or relatives to help you). The blanket should be kept over the pot as a tent and brought up and down, so that the steam crowds under the blanket and your lower back and thighs sweat profusely for ten minutes. Then carefully remove the blanket and the pan before thoroughly drying the sweaty areas. It is recommended remaining indoors for an hour after the steam bath and staying away from draughts.

If there's no one to help you, then lie face down and cover your lower back with five blankets for ten minutes, so that your waist can sweat profusely.

You can have a steam bath every three days, and not more often, because you will get exhausted. It is recommended for people suffering from cold-flu, back pain, lower back pain, shoulder periarthritis, tendonitis, hip-knee osteoarthritis, snakebite and intoxication from food-drugs-alcohol.

Shower, sitz baths

In cases of a sprained ankle, musculoskeletal disorders (MSDs), prostatic hypertrophy and haemorrhoids the use of alternating hot and cold tap water is beneficial. Using your bathtub shower handset, direct the water spray towards the affected areas. Apply cold water for twenty seconds, then hot water for five seconds. Keep switching the water temperature for a total of ten minutes, and finish with cold water. You can repeat this process even six times a day. If suffering from haemorrhoids or prostate hypertrophy, you should direct the water flow towards the anal and urogenital orifices respectively. You should use warm water, instead of hot, if you are dealing with haemorrhoids.

In cases of haemorrhoidal disease, you can alternate between sitting in two large water-filled washtubs. Both of them should have side handles, so that you may support yourself. The first should have very cold water (you could use ice cubes) and the second lukewarm. Start with the cold water washtub, sit in it for 20 seconds, and then switch to the one with the lukewarm water for about 5 seconds. The total duration of this process should be ten minutes. If it alleviates your discomfort, you may repeat the process six times a day.

Patients with gynecological problems (women's abdomens are more sensitive to cold), or sensitivity to cold water shouldn't use cold water.

SECTION 5: SELF ACUPUNCTURE

Introduction

Reading a book, regardless how well it is written, you can neither become a physician nor an acupuncturist.

You must always keep in mind that if you decide, on your own responsibility, to heal yourself by acupuncture, you should be getting better. If not, then you should contact your physician or the nearest medical doctor. If you decide to acupuncture yourself or your family the responsibility will be all yours.

I offer an alternative therapeutic perspective for people whose access to a medical doctor is too difficult or don't get better with conventional medical treatment and cannot afford to visit a private acupuncturist or for those who are open minded and assume responsibility for themselves. Unfortunately acupuncture is currently not applied to many public hospitals or it is applied only for pain.

Acupuncture is a safe therapeutical method if it is applied the way I describe. On the last page you will find the index of the acupuncture points.

The accompanying video with detailed demonstration of the self acupuncture technique (using one or two hands) and acupuncture points can be watched at http://youtu.be/358XNqIVPoc

Definition

Acupuncture is an ancient healing method based on the insertion of special fine needles into specific points on the body to regulate the flow of energy. The term acupuncture was coined by Jesuit missionaries in Beijing, and comes from the Latin words acus (pin, needle) and punctura (sting).

History

It is believed that carved, sharp edged stones called bian were used for acupuncture in China during the Stone Age. In 1963 a bian 4.5cm in length and dated from about 10,000 to 4,000 years was found in excavations in Mongolia. Shan-Hai-Jin (a geographical book which was written around 2000 years ago) states that jade suitable for the construction of stone needles can be found in the Kaou mountains. The use of needles is also described in Shuo-Wen-Chic-Chi (a book of similar chronology).

Needles from bamboo, animal bones, fish bones, pottery, porcelain, copper, brass, iron, silver and gold are also described in various later texts.

Today stainless needles are commonly used in acupuncture, sterilized in exactly the same way as syringes. They are very thin, flexible and unbreakable.

The oldest acupuncture book (about 300 BC) is Nei King (book of medicine) which is about a discourse of the Yellow Emperor (2697-2596 BC) with his six ministers of Health. In Nei King the theory of energy, acupuncture points, meridians (energy channels), the law of five elements (wood, fire, earth, metal, water), the 8 rules (yin-yang, interior-exterior, cold-heat, excess-deficiency), the diagnosis based on examination of pulses, the color of tongue and face, and the treatment techniques to stimulate and disperse using nine types of needles are fully examined.

In the 17th century Europeans were informed about acupuncture through traders and missionaries. The diplomatic trip of President Nixon in 1971 in China played an important role in the propagation of acupuncture in the West. A member of the journalistic mission, editor of the New York Times James Reston was surgically treated for acute appendicitis and acupuncture was used for postoperative analgesia.

Until recently acupuncture has been treated with disbelief and a rejection tendency by Western medical doctors as it is based on a philosophical structure totally different from the western medical thinking and the available literature sources are believed to lack credibility.

Signs of use of a similar method in Central Europe 5200 years ago have also been found. The 50 tattoos found on the acupuncture points of the Mummy Otzi (discovered in the glaciers of the Alps) is believed to have served therapeutic purposes.

In Ancient Hellas, according to mythology, the teacher of Asclepius (the mythical god of health) was Centaur Chiron. The two words Centaur Chiron in ancient Hellenic language are translated as embroider (sting) the aura (external energy of the body) with hands. Given that mythology is coded texts, then it is safe to believe that acupuncture was widely used in Ancient Hellas.

In the villages of the Valtou (southeast region of Artas district and north central region of Aitoloakarnanias district) which in the 16th century formed a county with Amfilochia as capital, they still traditionally use thermoacupuncture. In order to relieve pain, they place the edge of a red-hot wire, one centimeter above the skin area where the patient hurts, especially above joints, without touching the skin. For this reason many older women have signs of multiple small, round burns in their skin.

Basic Principles

The needles are placed mainly in 361 specific points of the body, which are called acupuncture points and which are arranged along intangible channels, the meridians (12 primary and 8 auxiliary).

The acupuncture points are three-dimensional, their shape is round or oval with a size of 3mm to 2,7cm and in the center are crossed by the meridians. Usually these points contain much more neurotransmitter substances and hormones than the surrounding tissues, such as acetylcholine, met-enkephalin, beta-endorphin, corticotropin hormone, cholokystokinin, norepinephrine, serotonin, gamma-aminobutyric acid, dopamine, dynorphin, prostaglandin E1 and vasomotor peptide. In addition atrial natriuretic peptide was found in the acupuncture points of Heart Meridian, while gastrin was found in Stomach Meridian.

Acupuncture points are distinguished from their specific position, but also by the following properties compared to the surrounding tissues:

1st Lower electrical resistance (10 kilo-ohms at the center point and 3 mega-ohms at the surrounding skin).

2nd Greater density of free nerve endings and sensory receptors and larger number of Meissner particles.

3rd Increased local temperature (P <0,001).

4th Significantly higher concentration of calcium ions.

5th Most are trigger points.

The Meridians according to Chinese energy theory are channels where energy constantly flows and the disruption of this flow causes disease. Energy can be compared to cars driven on alleys, streets, roads, avenues and highways (meridians). Energy is constantly flowing as cars are constantly moving on roads. Acupuncture points are found at the crossroads and at highway intersections. When disease occurs, it means that energy flow disorder happens. Usually there is excess and congestion of energy similar to excess of cars and traffic jam. By placing a needle in the appropriate acupuncture point-intersection is like placing an imaginary traffic warden to divert energy-cars to the air out of the body. The cars are not diverted to narrow streets but to huge air highways and the traffic jam-energy congestion (disease) is being cured.

In developed countries a disease rarely occurs because of energy deficit. Some roads, avenues, highways are empty, the needle (traffic warden) is placed at the beginning of the roads and allows energy (cars) to be transported via air in empty highways (meridians). The needle acts as a wise energy pipe between the skin (acupuncture points) and air. Depending on where there is more energy, the pipe (needle) transfers energy to the side where there is less energy.

The problem for scientists is what kind of energy is flowing in our body. Is it electric? Is it magnetic? Is it electromagnetic? Is it nuclear? What is it? How can we measure the energy so as to be sure that can we influence it?

Unfortunately the answers to these questions do not exist. Perhaps there is another form of energy beyond what we know.

This energy is vibrational in nature and it is not only in humans but also in everything that exists and has mass and matter (animals, plants, stones). The air also has this energy; we immediately understand the difference between the air of the polluted city center and the air in a wooded mountain.

Perhaps this energy also exists in minimum quantities in the black holes of space. This energy is a parallel event of the matter. I call it "Paralyli".

To understand the nature of the vibrational energy think of a calm lake in the center of which a stone drops. Immediately concentric circles are created that reach even the most distant points of the lake. One molecule stimulates the other and thus all the molecules of the lake receive the effect of the stimulus which in this case is the stone.

Proportionally, man is the lake and the stones are the emotions as well as the external effects (cold, heat, wind, nutrition, exercise, electromagnetic, solar and cosmic radiation etc.).

Energy flows in channels which are divided in Primary Meridians and in auxiliary channels.

Each Primary Meridian consists of 10 vibrational "fibers". When yang rises in Primary Meridians (in symptomatic or not symptomatic disease), then the intervals between fibers are reduced. Fibers "seem" to unite and the Primary Meridians seems smaller. The opposite happens when yin increases. The intervals are increased, fibers can be clearly seen and the Meridians seem bigger.

According to the Chinese energy theory, the human organs which are protected deeply in the body maintain the energetic essence and through the meridians they regulate the spiritual-mental and physical health.

Acupuncture influences the meridians which are directly related to the energy state of the human body and thus catalytically influences human health.

The needles used are usually sterile, disposable and made of stainless steel. There are also bronze, silver and golden needles.

Acupuncture needles are much smaller than needles of syringes used in routine clinical practice. Their thickness (diameter) is usually between 0,20 mm and 0,40 mm. Their length varies and depends on the installation site. In each session the needles are inserted for about 30 minutes.

Indications of acupuncture
(according to the World Health Organization,
http://tcm.health-info.org/WHO-treatment-list.htm # _treat)

Diseases, symptoms or conditions for which acupuncture has proved through controlled trials to be an effective treatment:

Allergic rhinitis, headache, nausea, vomiting, side effects of radiotherapy and chemotherapy, rheumatoid arthritis, correction of embryo position, biliary and renal colic, hypotension, hypertension, neck pain, depression, toothache, dysentery, knee pain, shoulder periarthritis, dysmenorrhea, leucopenia, postoperative pain, epigastric pain, back pain, sciatica, sprain, stroke, facial pain, labor induction and epikondylitis.

Diseases, symptoms or conditions for which the therapeutic effect of acupuncture has been shown but for which further proof is needed:

Gastroenteritis, alcoholism, facial palsy, bronchial asthma, cancer pain, cholecystitis, cholelithiasis, closed head injury, non-insulin dependent diabetes, earache, epistaxis, epidemic hemorrhagic fever, ofthalmalgia, female infertility, fibromyalgia, gastrointestinal motor disorders, herpes zoster, post-herpes pain, dyslipidemia, viral status in hepatitis B, insomnia, labor pain, lactation deficiency, male sexual dysfunction non-organic, Menière disease, detox from drugs and smoking, postoperative recovery, pruritus, neurodermatitis, osteoarthritis, obstructive vascular pain, recurrent urinary tract infections, obesity, polycystic syndrome, chronic prostatitis, reflex sympathetic dystrophy, traumatic urinary retention, stiff neck, urolithiasis, Sjogren syndrome, schizophrenia, vascular dementia, syndrome Tietze, sore throat (including tonsilitis), ulcerative colitis, whooping cough and drug induced sialism.

Diseases, symptoms or conditions for which there are only individual controlled trials reporting some therapeutic effects, but for which acupuncture is worth trying because treatment by conventional and other therapies is difficult:

Chloasma, deafness, neuropathic bladder in spinal cord injury, central serous choroeidopathy, hypofreneia, chronic pulmonary heart disease, color blindness, irritable colon syndrome and small airway obstruction.

Diseases, symptoms or conditions for which acupuncture may be tried provided the practitioner has special modern medical knowledge and adequate monitoring equipment:

Coma, diarrhea in infants and children, infant convulsions, breathlessness in chronic obstructive pulmonary disease, viral encephalitis, coronary disease and progressive bulbar and pseudo-bulbar palsy.

German nationwide study

In 2001 Germany started a nationwide study on acupuncture and its effect on tension headache, migraine, chronic back pain and knee osteoarthritis. It lasted 4 years, it required 7 million euro paid from public insurance funds and involved 7,300 medical doctors-acupuncturists and 43,000 patients.

The first phase consisted of 10 acupuncture sessions over a period of 5 weeks to 40,000 people. The 89,9% felt improvement in their complaints, 50,7% of which in the first 4 acupuncture sessions. There were no deaths; there were less than 1% total faints and mild local inflammation. This phase was preliminary and did not include a control sample.

Because there was success, it was followed by the second phase. Prospective randomized controlled study compared acupuncture with conventional medical treatment and fake acupuncture.

The study proved that acupuncture had significantly better results in back pain and osteoarthritis in the knee and the same results in tension headache and migraine. The results cited in 4 papers published in recognized international medical journals:

Brinkhaus B et al. University Medical Center, Berlin, Germany.
Acupuncture in patients with chronic low back pain: A Randomized Controlled trial.
Archives of Internal Medicine 2006 Feb 27; 166 (4):450-7.

Witt C et al. University Medical Center, Berlin, Germany.

Acupuncture in Patients with Osteoarthritis of the Knee: A Randomized Trial.

Lancet 2005 Jul 9-15; 366 (9480):136-43.

Diener HC et al. Department of Neurology, University Essen, Germany.

Efficacy of acupuncture for the prophylaxis of migraine: a multicentre randomized controlled clinical trial.

Lancet Neurology 2006 Apr; 5 (4):310-6.

Melchart D et al. Centre for Complementary Medicine Research, Department of Internal Medicine II, Technische Universität München, Kaiserstr 9, 80801 Munich, Germany.

Acupuncture in patients with tension-type headache: randomized controlled trial.

British Medical Journal 2005 Aug 13; 331 (7513):376-82.

After the above mentioned nationwide study (although it remains unknown how acupuncture acts) the Central German Health Council recognized acupuncture as a scientific treatment for chronic back pain and osteoarthritis of the knee and proposed the approval of acupuncture by the public insurance funds (18/4/2006). The German Ministry of Health ratified the above proposal (09/19/2006).

Types of needles, cost and where to find them

The acupuncturists use industrial stainless steel needles which are disposable and sterilized with an internationally approved method.

Nowadays an acupuncturist rarely uses needles multiple times (the patient purchases and keeps the needles which the acupuncturist each time sterilizes). I disagree with this method because, except from the infection risk, the used needles are energy charged and they will function less even on the same patient. The needles are cheap and it is not worth reusing them.

I buy disposable needles, image 4, with a guide tube (so that the needle penetrates easily, painlessly and in a concrete depth of half a centimeter) from the importer Skouras Vasilios (19 Skoufa street, Kolonaki, Athens, Hellas tel: 00302103637373, 00306934698693).

I use needles 0,20 x 13mm (short) for acupuncture points located on the head and fingers, and needles 0,30 x 75mm (long) for the other acupuncture points. The guide tube is a cylindrical plastic tube that surrounds the sized 0,5cm longer needle and helps the needle to penetrate in the particular 0,5cm depth without bending.

A box of needles usually contains 100 needles at a total cost of around 6 euros. There are more expensive needles from gold, silver and copper.

In Hellas, both in peace and especially in war times, when there is lack of pharmaceutical material, we can apply acupuncture using needles from plants (aspalathos, lemon tree, acacia, wild pear tree, pomegranate, farnasian acacia, pyracantha) which are plentiful in the Hellenic nature. In Hellas one of the most frequently found shrub is aspalathos (official Latin name calycotome villosa), images 2 and 3. Aspalathos is also called sfylachti (in the region of Aitoloakarnania) or sfalachtro (in the region of Messinia) or asfalachtos or asfelachtos or spalathos or spalathros or spalachtri. In Cyprus it is called spalathia, asparagkathia, asporracho, arkorracho.

It is a thorny shrub with trifoliate leaves, short stalks and yellow flowers in spring. Ordo: Fabales, Familia: Fabaceae, Subfamilia: Faboideae, Tribus: Genisteae, Genus: Calicotome.

Aspalathos is self sown and in my humble opinion has a much better effect than industrial needles because of the juice that it contains.

Currently it is used as firewood (where there are no forests) and as natural hedge. Dioscurides wrote that Gods punished the tyrants in hell with aspalathos's branches.

A prerequisite to thorn needles is not to break when they penetrate the skin. The needles from cactus are unsuitable for acupuncture because they both break and irritate.

Thorn needles are more effective than industrial-type steel needles because of the contained juices. The crucial disadvantage is that the industrial needles are sterile, while the thorn needles can not be sterilized. A few decades ago we used to walk in wild nature or in villages and did not bother us if we got pinched by various thorns or if we got scratches. Nowadays mothers have antiseptics in their bags and children apply iodine on each and every tiny scratch.

If you are not afraid to take responsibility for yourselves without asking the physician (who is trained to demand everything to be sterile) to give you guarantees, you can use thorn needles. Choose thorns from the part of the plant which is more protected (i.e. that cannot be reached by the urine of a dog) and sterilize their sharp end with alcohol.

For people without access to industrial-type needles, or to thorns, an alternative solution is the large fish bones; if you want a sterile needle, then use insulin needles.

If you are afraid to insert needles, then one solution is to place little magnet stickers on the acupuncture points. The results will be much poorer and the purchase is much more expensive. Let the magnets on for one hour and then throw them away. Avoid using them again or in the evenings. The placement of magnets on acupuncture points is called magnetic acupuncture. Magnet stickers are supplied by Skouras Vasilios who is located at 19 Skoufa street, Kolonaki, Athens, tel: 00302103637373, 00306934698693. Magnet stickers are also sold in many pharmacies. Magnetic acupuncture is easily applied to children who react negatively to the sting of a needle.

Is acupuncture painful?

I will never forget the answer of a young man addicted to heroin, when I offered helping him with acupuncture. He was in deprivation syndrome and said "no, I am afraid that it will be painful", even though his body was over pinched by syringes.

The classic question that almost all patients do before the first acupuncture is "Doctor, is it painful?"

The answer is: No. Acupuncture is painless.

There are a few acupuncture points on the fingertips and soles which are not painless, but pain is instant and much less compared to the pain caused by the syringe when blood is drawn.

Of course the technique is very important; the more experienced the acupuncturist is, the less pain. The secret is the needle to penetrate very quickly the skin-epidermis and enter into the subcutaneous space. The skin consists of the outer skin, the epidermis which has many nerve endings responsible for pain sensation and the inner skin, the subcutaneous, which is soft because of the fat.

Technique

The acupuncture needles which I use have a guide tube (plastic tube). The needle is immobilized in the guide tube by a small triangular plastic safety lock, image 4. The needle consists of a. the head which is thick, cylindrical and steel, b. the body which is thinner flexible steel and c. the top which is more thin, unbreakable and sharp edged so as to easily penetrate the skin. The guide tube is half a centimeter smaller in length than the needle.

Acupuncture using two hands

Remove the needle from its packaging which keeps it sterile. Those of you who are right-handed hold with your left hand the plastic tube in a horizontal position with the head of the needle towards the right side of your body. Then with your right hand remove the triangular plastic safety that immobilizes the needle in the tube and throw it away (recycle it). Now grab with the right thumb and index finger simultaneously the head of the needle and the edge (towards the head of the needle) of the guide tube.

Place the other edge of the guide tube at the acupuncture point (the skin at that point must be free of dirt, totally clean) and hold with your left thumb and index finger on the center of the guide tube. Release your right fingers. With the left fingers on the center of the tube, press the guide tube towards the skin, image 28. Abruptly tap the head of the needle with your right index finger. You must feel the skin of your index finger touching the edge of the guide tube so as the needle to penetrate one half a centimeter in the skin. There are a few acupuncture points where the skin is very thin. At these points the index finger will not touch the edge of the guide tube and the needle will penetrate only two or three mm.

Remove the guide tube; you are now a self acupuncturist.

Acupuncture using one hand

Grab simultaneously the head of the needle and the edge of the guide tube (you have removed the plastic safety) with the thumb and the middle finger. Place the other edge of the tube at the acupuncture point. Slide the two fingers on the guide tube for about one centimeter or less if the needle is short. Then press the tube towards the skin and abruptly tap with your index finger, image 29. Remove the guide tube, the needle has been inserted.

How to avoid side effects

In order to avoid fainting during acupuncture treatment you must be lying down and be calm. Do not change position especially with abrupt movements so as not to press the needles unintentionally.

In order to avoid subcutaneous hematomas or bruises, do not place the guide tubes on skin areas where are visible blood vessels under the surface. Of course, in case some bleeding occurs you must not panic; just press the bleeding point. Remember that the physicians put large catheters into big vessels and when they take them out, they press the entry point to stop the bleeding. So when there is bleeding over or under the skin surface (you see edema or bruise) press the point with cotton for 2 minutes and the bleeding or the enlargement of the edema-bruise will stop.

If there is a clotting problem (e.g. when patient takes anticoagulants), then you need to press for more time or use a moderately tight elastic bandage (not to cause problems in blood supply) and leave it for 10 minutes.

If the blood perfusion of a region or a limb is problematic (e.g. diabetic angiopathy) do not insert needles at this region or limb.

Be careful; never place needles without the guide tube which I use. Needles should never be inserted deeper than one centimeter. Serious complications from needles inserted deeply are reported in the literature. For example, paraplegia was caused because a needle was inserted in the spine 10cm deeply or pneumothorax from a needle inserted in the chest 5cm deeply.

Be careful; it is forbidden to insert needles on sexual organs, i.e. testes, penis, urethra, vulva (pudenda, clitoris and lips) and vagina. It is also forbidden to insert needles on breasts, anus, lips, mouth, ear canal, eye and eyelids. It is allowed to insert needles only where there is skin and not in mucosa (e.g. tongue, nostrils) or nails.

Be careful; do not insert needles on pregnant women (risk of miscarriage) unless you are a qualified acupuncturist.

Be careful; it is forbidden to reuse the needle on another patient. I go one step further and say that the used needle should not be inserted into the same patient again. When a needle is used it is charged with energy. The preferable and more effective needle is the uncharged.

Finally, **be careful** not to accidentally get pinched from a used needle.

If you follow the above mentioned you may not have the perfect therapeutic effect but surely you will not have any side effects (the above mentioned or any medication induced ones) either. So it's safe to try self acupuncture.

Acupuncture rules and duration

Always at the beginning of a disease consult a physician.

The fewer needles you use, the better; usually not more than four.

If you want to turn off all the lights in a palace you shut down the general switch and you don't go to every room to turn off the lights.

You can insert a needle into every painful or itchy or annoying or numb point of your skin except the forbidden parts of the body.

If you forget the direction of a needle insert it perpendicularly.

If there is no obvious improvement with acupuncture treatment, consult a physician.

I leave the needles for half an hour as it has been said by extra-sensor healers that the circle of energy in the human body lasts 25 minutes. You can leave the needles more, 45 minutes or one hour if you feel better with them or if you face resistance when you try taking them out.

Often as time passes the needles come out of the skin by themselves because the energy drifts the needle when it comes out of the body. It is not wise to leave the needles for hours because the energy will be coming out and getting in constantly. Your body will get a little tired. If for some reason you forgot to remove the needle or you left the needle all night on purpose, it is not a big deal (i.e. if you suffered from insomnia, inserted a needle and at last you got asleep, you should not use the alarm clock to take out the needle in half an hour).

The precise time to remove a needle can be determined only by an acupuncturist who can feel the vibrations over the needle.

The waveform of the vibrations over the head of a needle which disperses energy (transfers energy to the air) is shown in the diagram, page 102. The perfect time to remove the needle is at time-point 1 and it is good to remove the needle at time-point 0, similarly at stimulation.

During acupuncture I recommend that you intentionally relax (the needles will also relax you). With your eyes closed, repeat silently and continuously a little prayer (i.e. God help me, or Lord Jesus Christ have mercy on me) and focus your mind on each word of the prayer. If you have other thoughts (something which always happens) do not try to delete them but re-focus on each word of the prayer.

During acupuncture you must not eat, chew, drink or smoke because all your energy should focus on your treatment. Lie in a quiet, relatively warm room (when motionless one gets cold easily) without telephones, television, or radio on and accept acupuncture as a gift to yourself that you rightly deserve.

It is better to do acupuncture during the day, because at night the energy goes into deeper layers of the body. Of course if you have a headache in the middle of the night you will do acupuncture and you will probably feel relieved.

Stimulating, dispersion

Stimulation means that energy from the atmosphere goes into our body through the needle. When you remove the needle you should simultaneously press gently, cover the acupuncture point for 3 seconds to "tap" the skin hole so as the energy does not leave the body and goes into the atmosphere.

Disperse means that energy from the body comes out to the atmosphere. When you remove the needle you should not press the acupuncture point because we want the energy to come out.

When you use thorn needles and your aim is dispersion, calycotome villosa (images 2 and 3) is the best choice. When you need stimulation, the thorns from a wild pear tree are the best choice even though they are bulkier and hurt a little more.

For encyclopedic reasons you should know that the needles of gold are most suitable for stimulation, while the needles of silver or copper or steel are suitable primarily for dispersion.

When stimulation is very important for the patient, after the acupuncturist has inserted the needle, he/she grasps the head of the needle with the thumb and index finger and for a few seconds transmits his/her energy to the patient. When one wants to transmit his/her energy, must be calm and dedicated. Repeating quietly the prayer "God help the patient" is very helpful when you transmit your energy.

In winter and especially for persons who generally feel their limbs cold, moxa combustion is helpful. Firstly I place a needle and then I heat the needle's head with burning moxa. Moxa is a plant which has the official Latin name artemisia vulgaris. Instead of moxa you can apply heat from burning coal or burning iron. You can see the resemblance with the red hot wire that was used in the Hellenic villages of Valtos.

Moxa is supplied by Skouras Vasilios (19 Skoufa street, Kolonaki, Athens, tel: 00302103637373, 00306934698693).

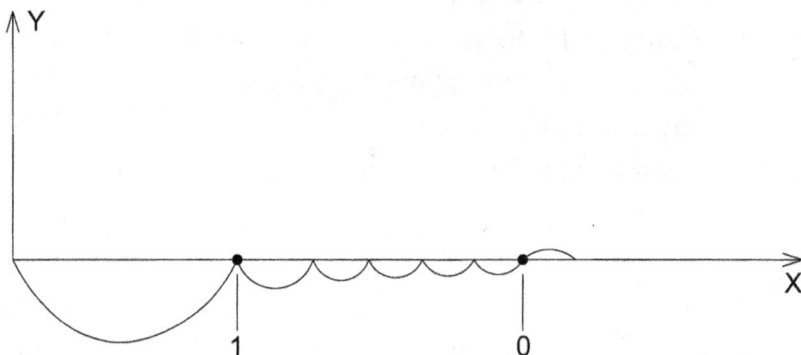

Stimulation waveform

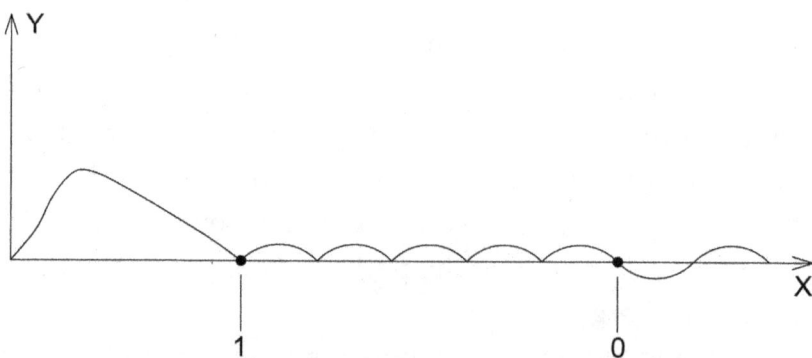

Dispersion waveform

Frequency

Acupuncture can be repeated daily until the acute phase of the disease is over.

If the symptoms become milder (usually within three days) then acupuncture can be applied every two days. If there is no obvious improvement, consult a physician again.

In Known chronic diseases acupuncture can be applied every three days for 3 months. Do a fifteen-day break and go on twice weekly and so forth.

In case of a severe pain or symptom acupuncture two and three times daily. When you acupuncture for detoxification of heroin, the first two days you can repeat acupuncture three and four times daily.

Each time, acupuncture takes about half an hour and is called acupuncture session.

Results

In many cases the effect of acupuncture is immediate (within the acupuncture session); sometimes the results are seen by the patient the next day and in chronic diseases, the results appear in a month. The patient should have improvement in a week except from chronic diseases.

Impressive results are seen in several conditions described in the following pages.

There are times when acupuncture does not help at all but fortunately it does not have side effects.

Hippocrates said that the best results occur when the patient really wants to get well (makes an effort: relaxes, exercises, watches their diet, does not smoke or drink etc.) and when their relatives, physician and also the stars (weather condition, prayers from known and unknown people, etc.) help.

In ancient China, except from acupuncture they used medicine herbs, cupping therapy, massage, immobilization of broken limbs and relaxation techniques. They considered physical activity, nutrition, rest and abuse prevention (drinking, sex, long trips) very important. The physicians were paid only by the healthy people.

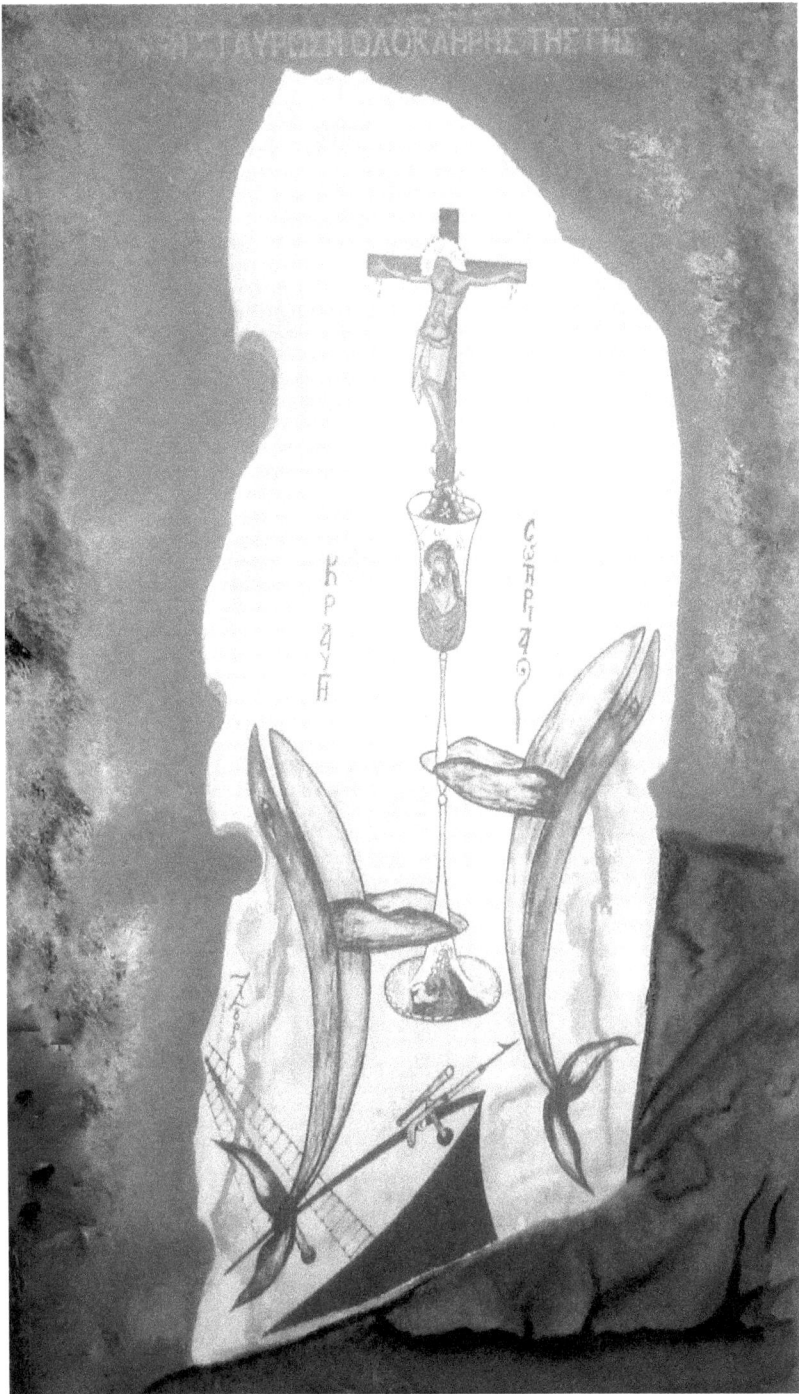

Image 1

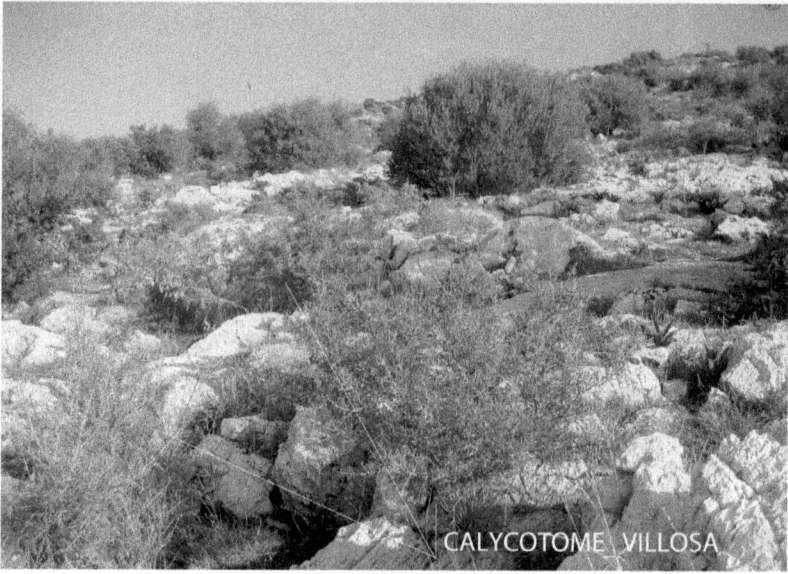

CALYCOTOME VILLOSA

Image 2

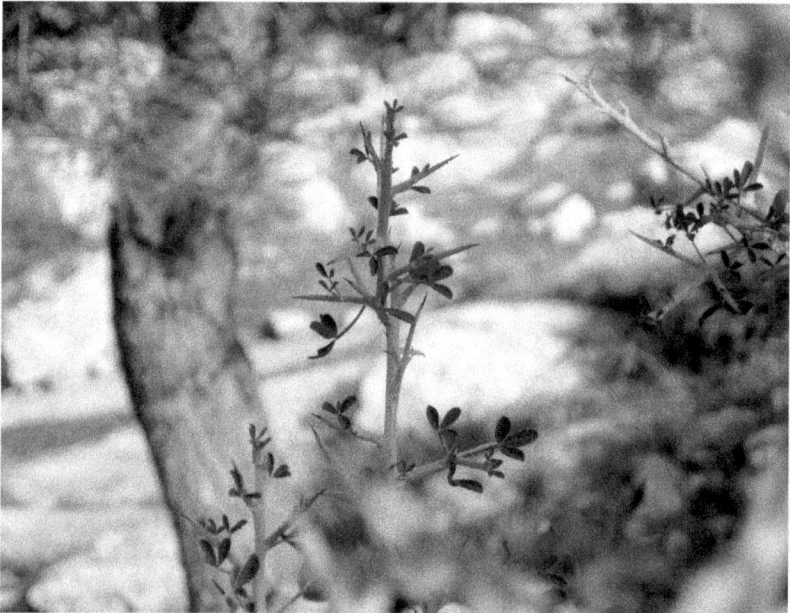

Image 3

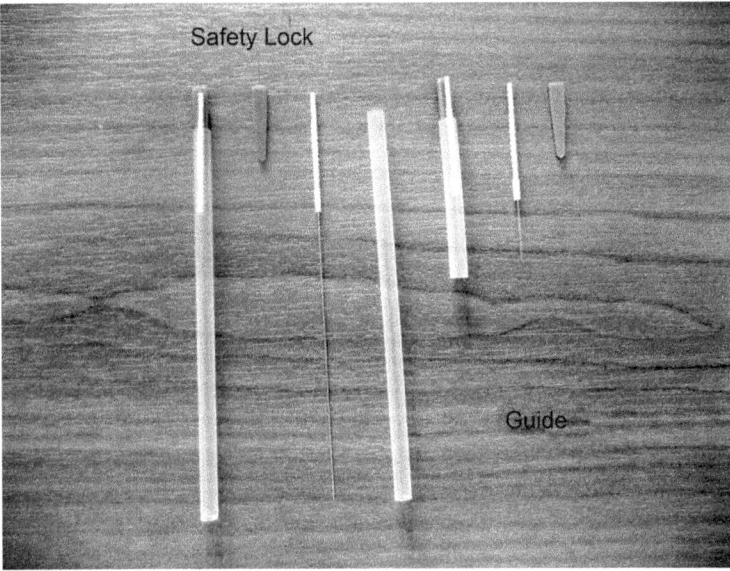

Image 4

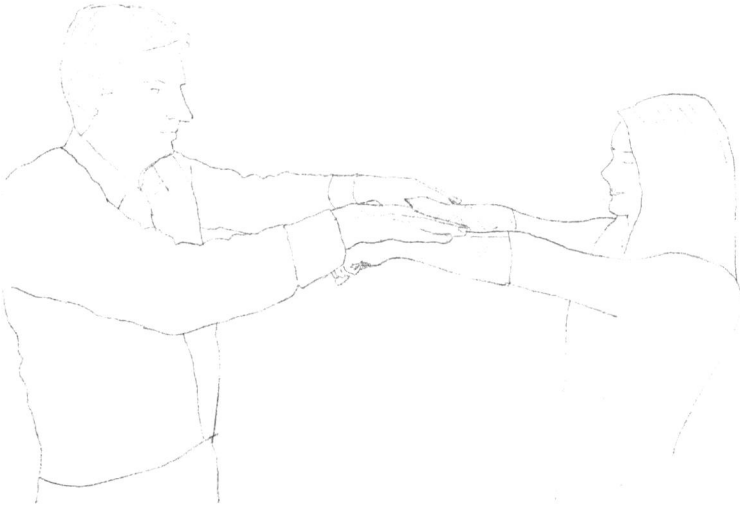

Image 5

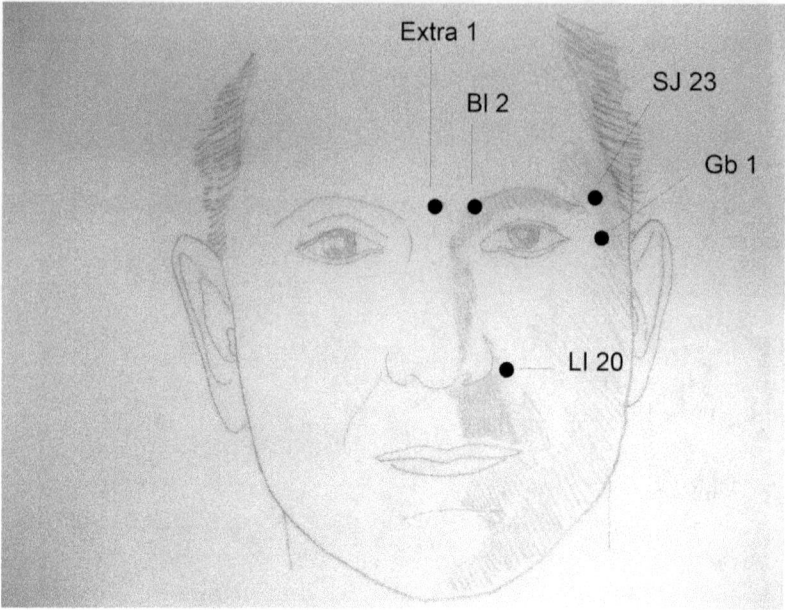

Image 6

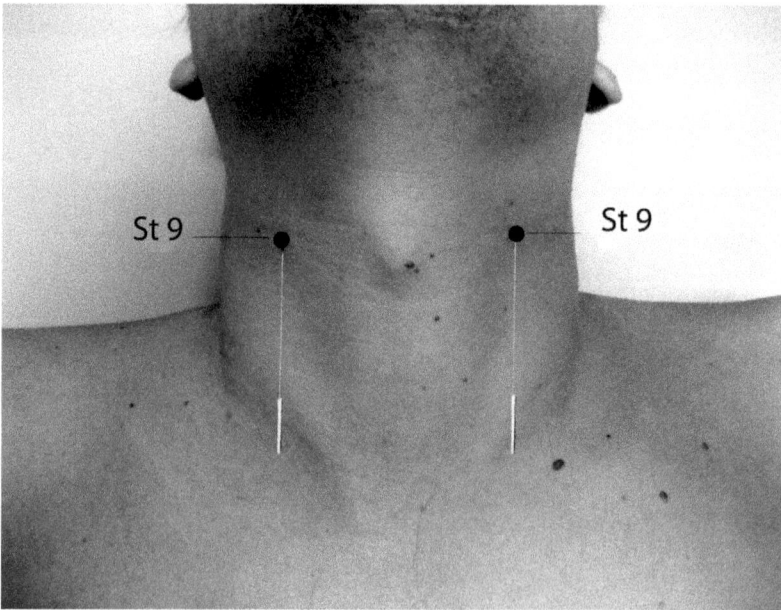

Image 7

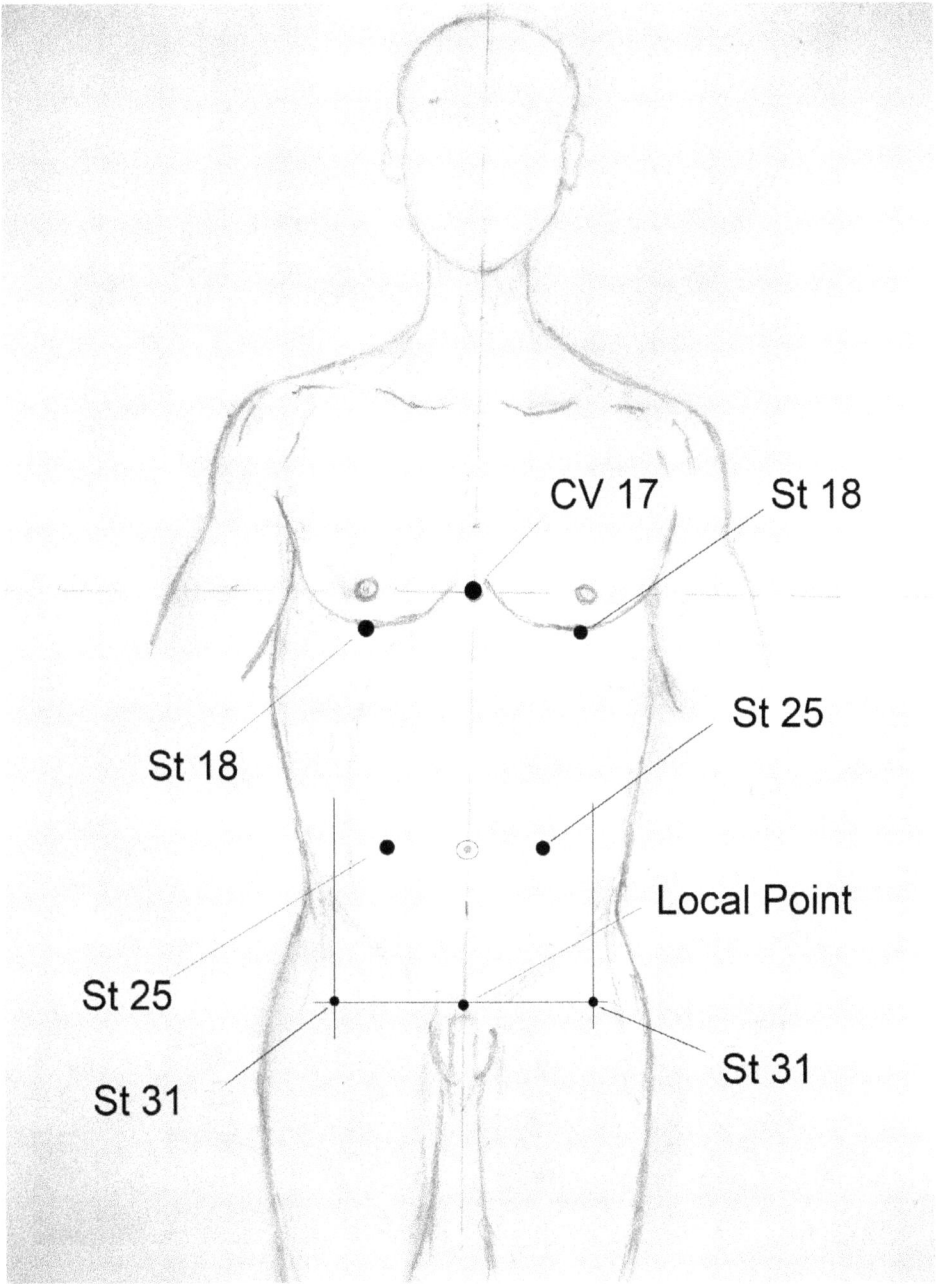

Image 8

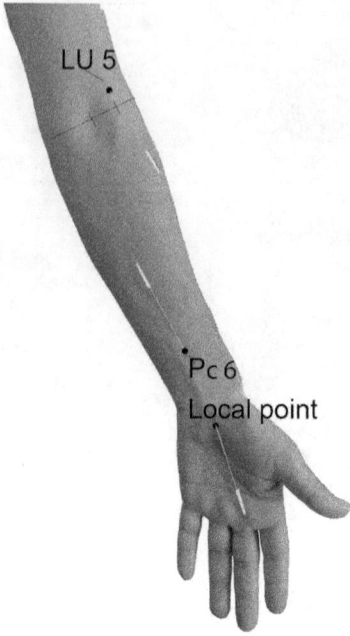

Image 9

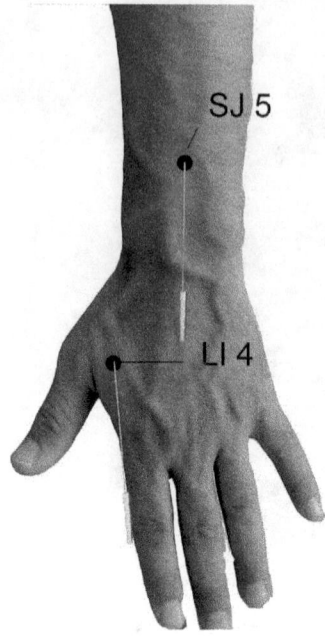

Image 10

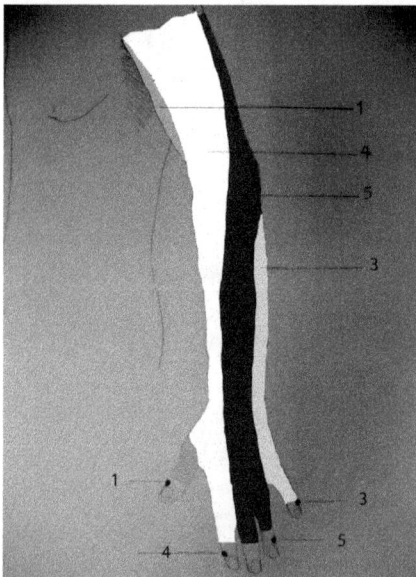

Image 11

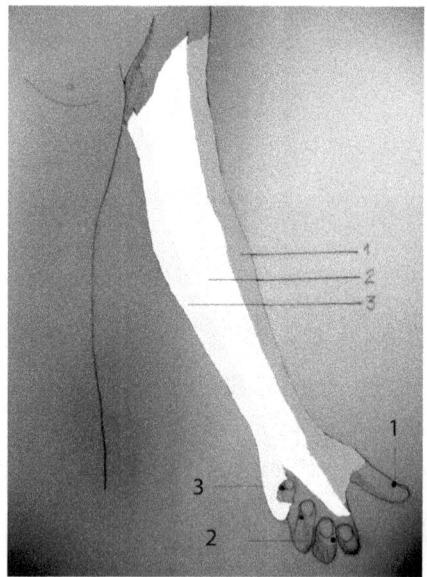

Image 12

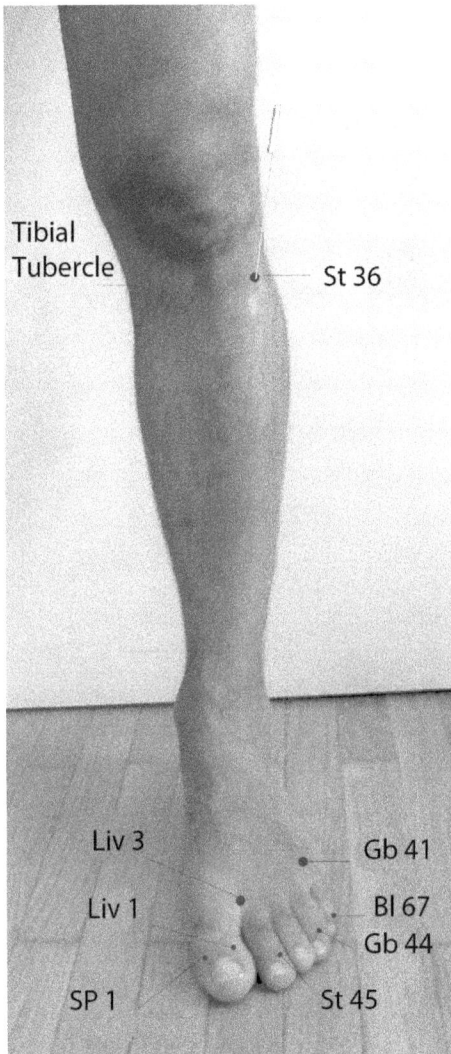

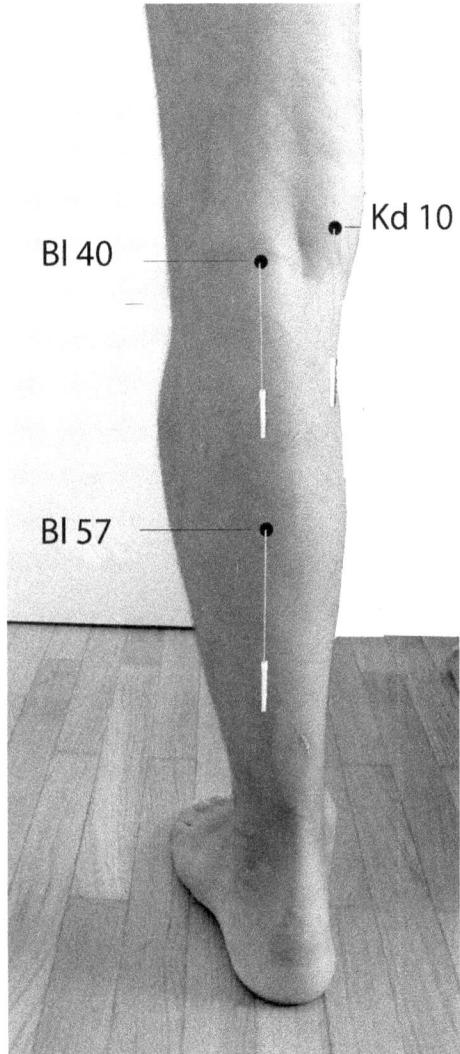

Image 13   Image 14

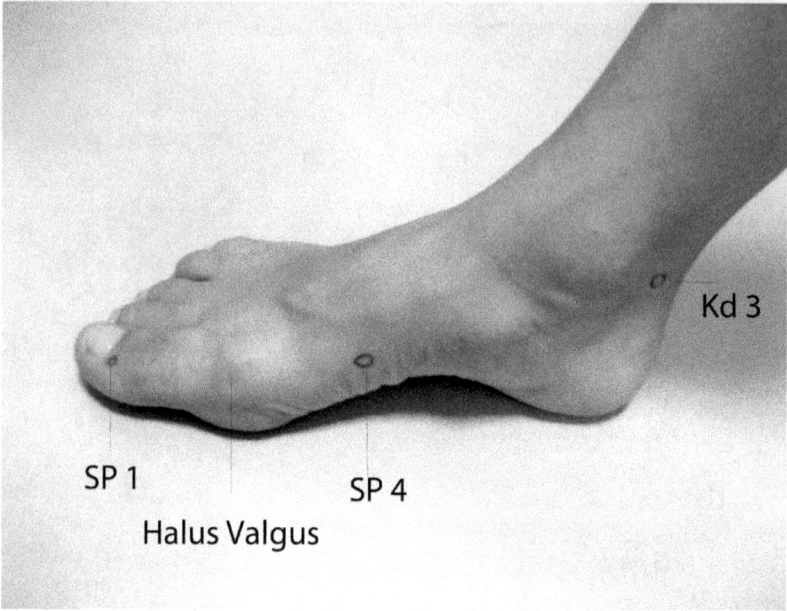

Image 15

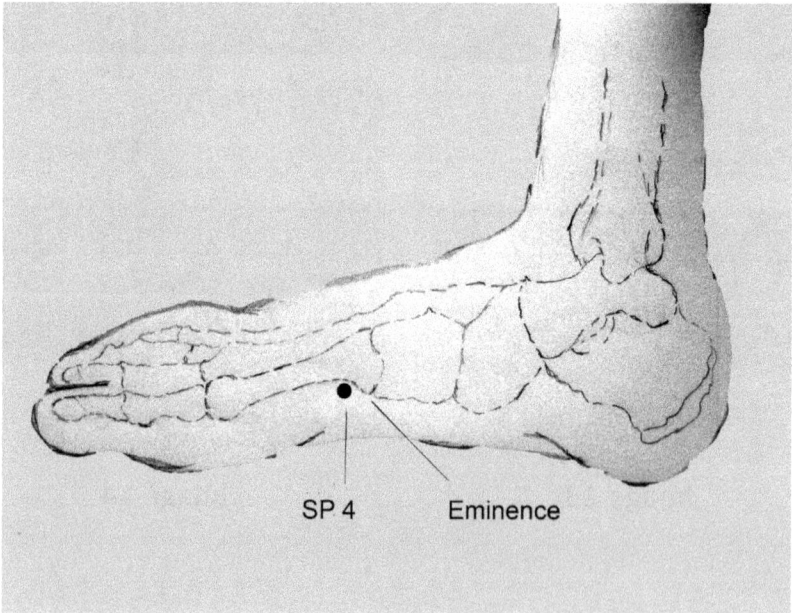

Image 16

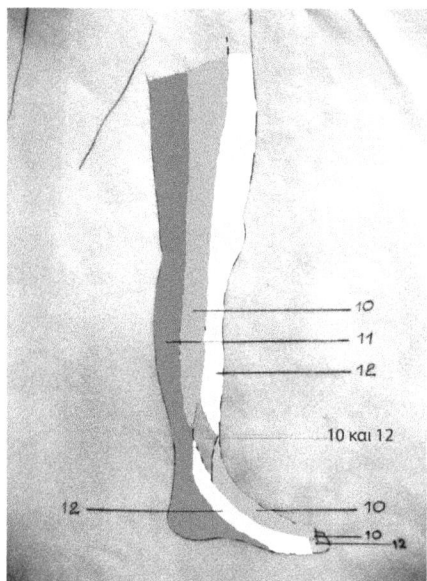

Image 17

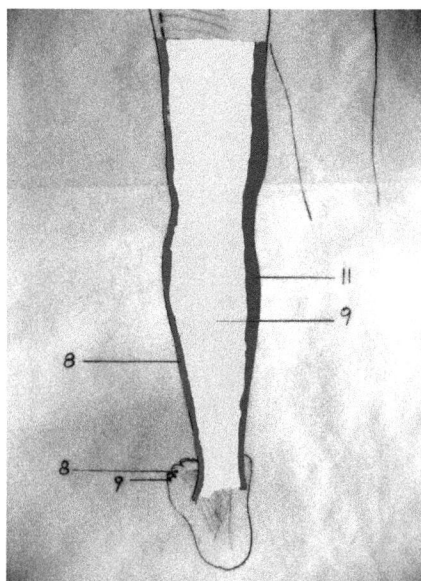

Image 18

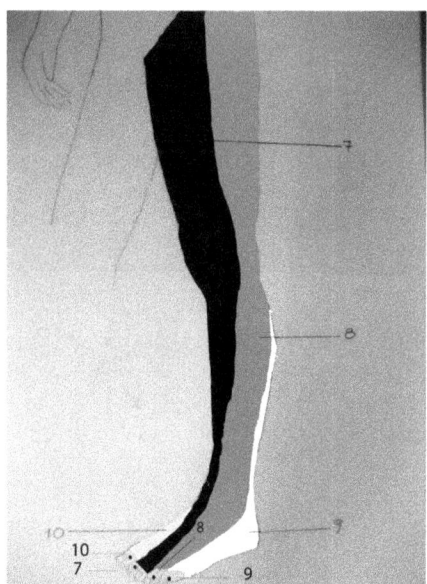

Image 19

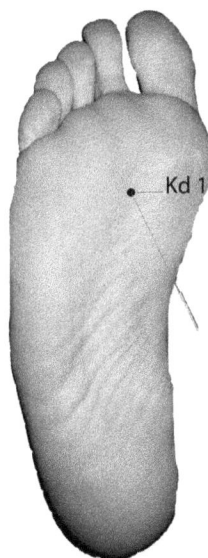

Image 20

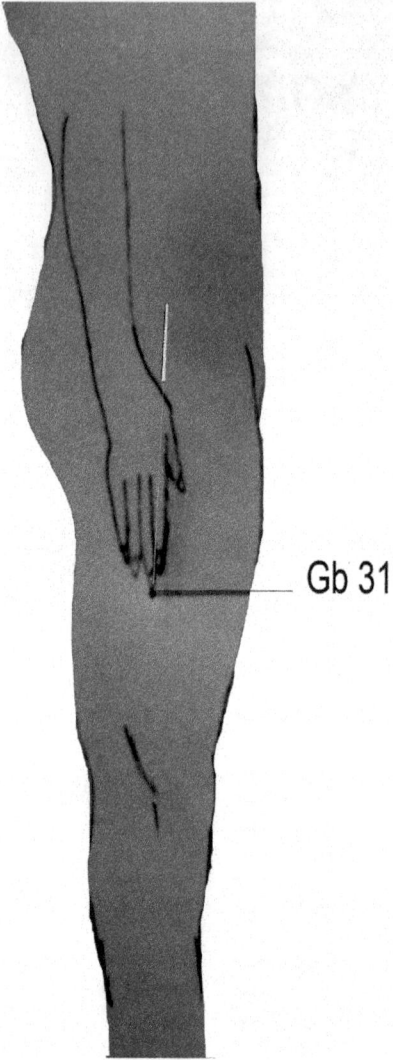

Gb 31

Image 21

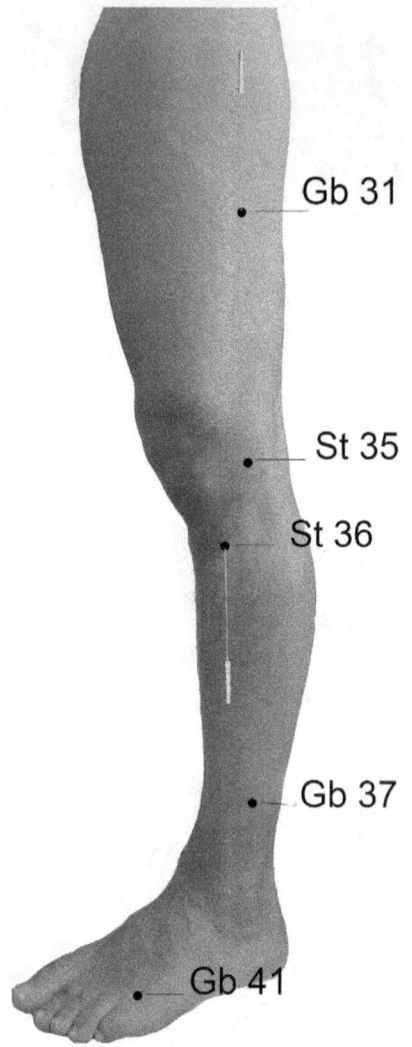

Gb 31

St 35

St 36

Gb 37

Gb 41

Image 22

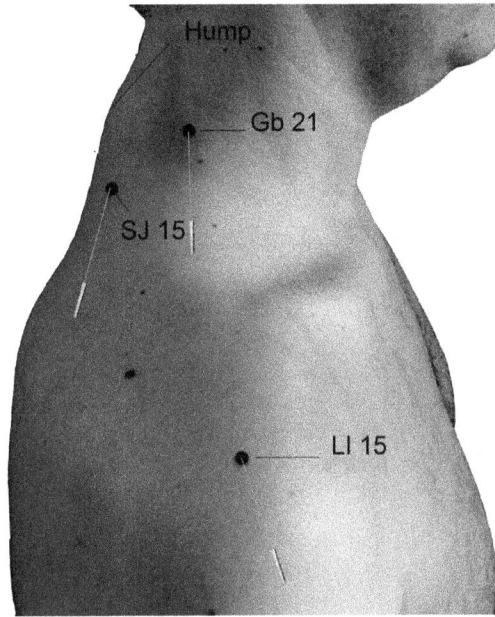

Image 23

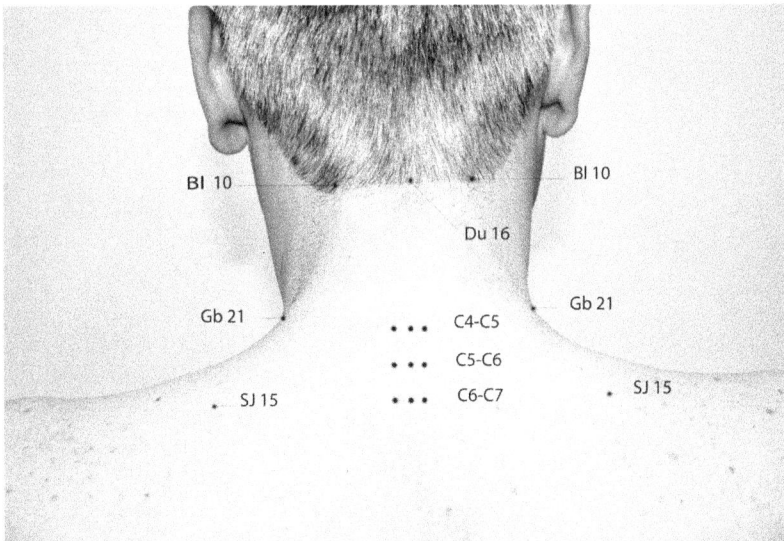

Image 24

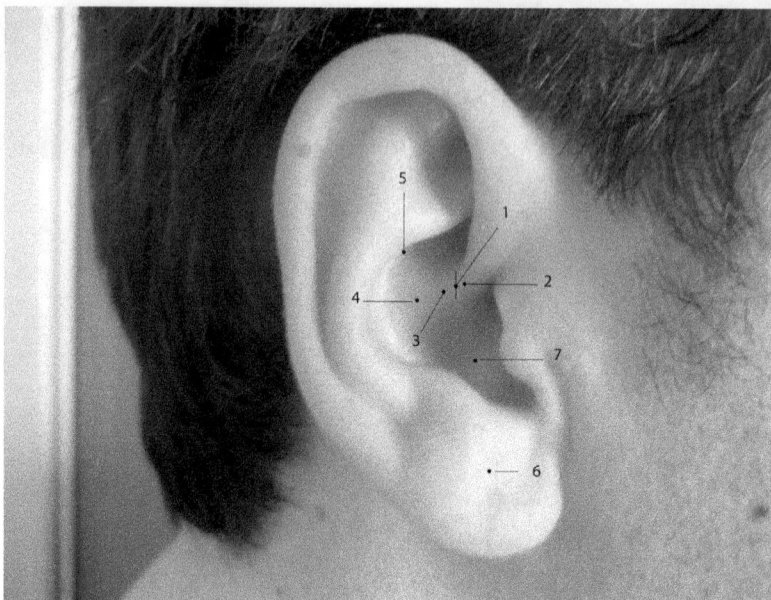

Image 25

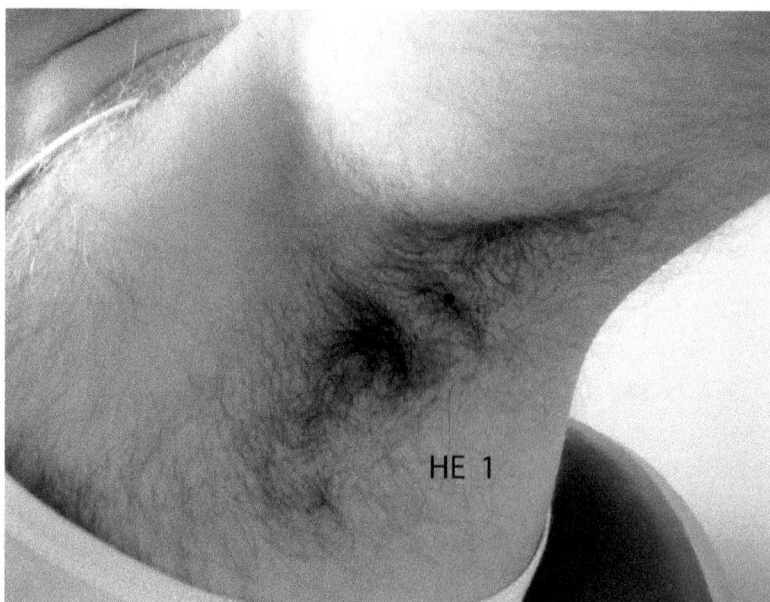

Image 26

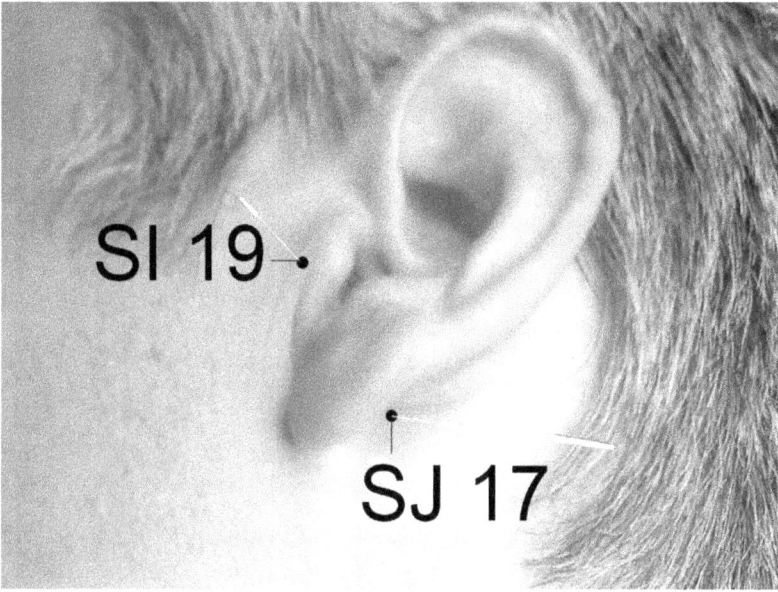

Image 27

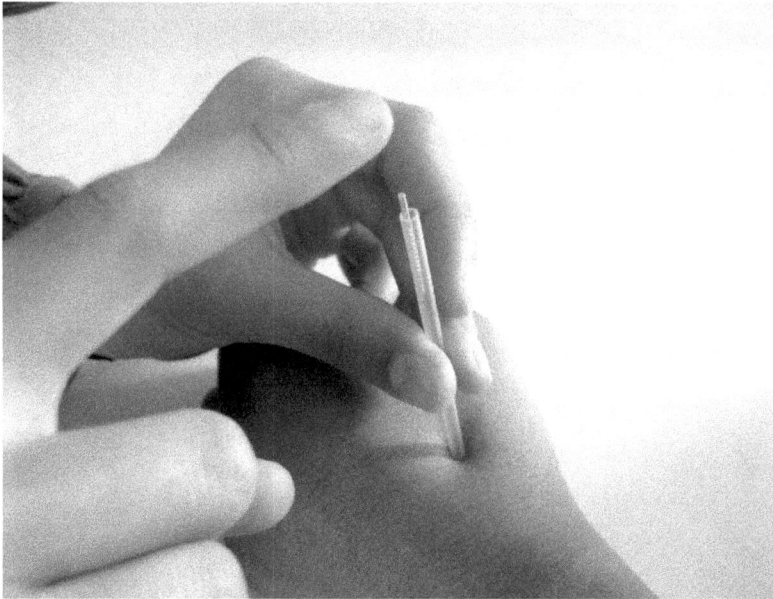

Image 28

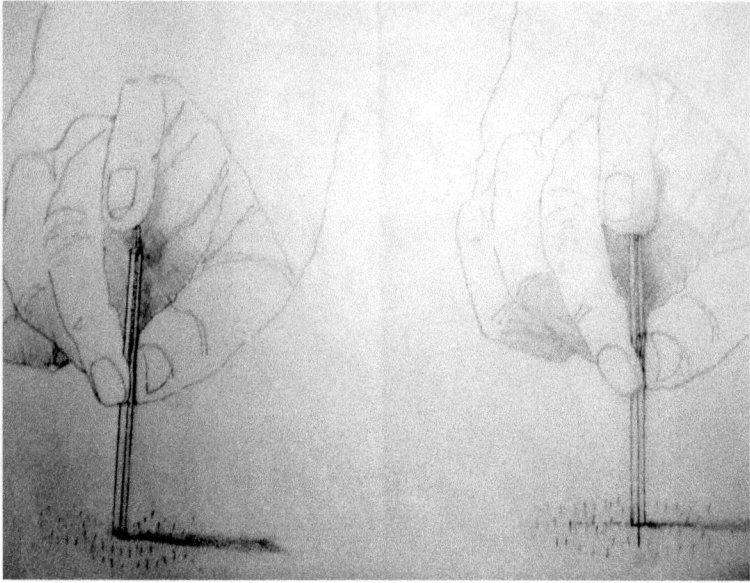

Image 29

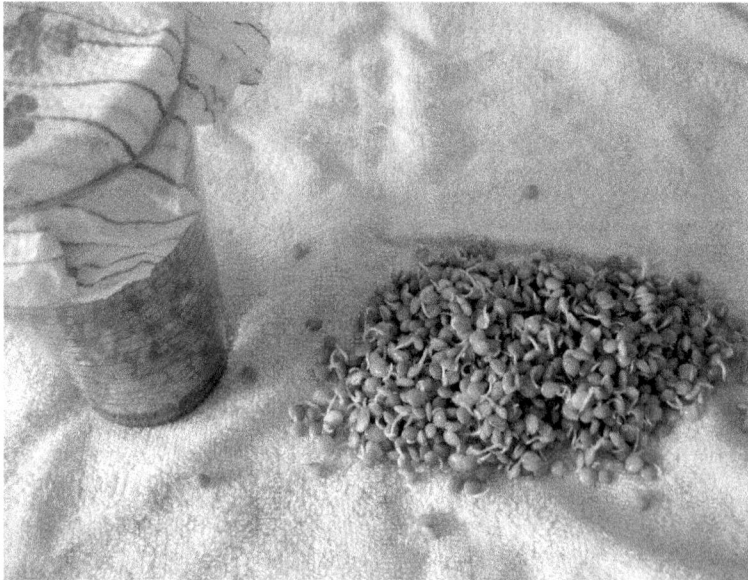

Image 30

Relaxation

The easiest and at the same time the most necessary self acupuncture is that for relaxation. In every patient I use needles for relaxation because in developed countries we all suffer from the scourge of the era, from stress.

Having, being or wanting result in anxiety or stress and of course stress adversely affects our well being.

Many patients say "I don't have anxiety, I am very calm" but the truth is that only some hermits on Mount Athos or some next door saints have no anxiety. They never visit physicians because they leave everything entirely to the Lord.

There are two types of stress, the daily and the deep stress.

Daily stress is the stress of the so-called simple things, e.g. having to catch up a bus or to cook well. In case of daily stress I insert a needle at point Extra 1, dispersion. This point is located at the intersection of the vertical midline of your body with the imaginary horizontal line joining the start of eyebrows, image 6. It is also called the third eye.

If stress causes headache on one side of the head, I choose the SJ 23 point, dispersion. This point is located in a hollow (like most acupuncture points) on the outer, upper edge of the eye orbit. To find this small hollow, slide the index finger over the eyebrow from the base of the nose (nasal root) towards the ear. The hollow is where the eyebrow ends and slightly to the ear, image 6.

At both points, Extra 1 and SJ 23, I insert the needle perpendicular to the skin. The day of a full moon, the previous and the next is better not to insert needles at these points. If it is necessary I leave the needle only 10 minutes. Sometimes when I take the needle out from these points blood comes out but stops easily with minimal (and should be minimal) pressure with a cotton ball. When blood comes out, it is an indication of full stress but it doesn't mean that there is no stress when blood doesn't come out.

At the end of a half hour the needle should come out very easily, if it doesn't, it means that is better to remove it later. Often, as time passes, the needle comes out by itself because when energy comes out of the body it drifts the needle.

Daily stress can appear as headache, pain in the cervical area, insomnia, tinnitus, dizziness, numbness, or as any other symptom. I remind you once again that when symptoms persist and there is no clear improvement or elimination of discomfort, the patient must consult a physician, do blood tests and imaging evaluation (x-ray, ultrasound, CT, MRI or angiography etc.).

Deep stress is caused by an important reason as divorce, death of a beloved person, problematic relationship with the boss at work, etc. . Symptoms that characterize deep stress-anxiety may be similar to those of daily stress but are usually more intense. Often they are similar to those of depression, i.e. insomnia, fatigue, apathy, emotionalism or sometimes they are manifested as a tendency to eat more, alcoholism, smoking, drugs, sexual perversion and self-destruction.

In this case I choose point Pc 6, stimulation. It is located in the midline of the anterior surface of the forearm, approximately 5cm above the wrist, between the tendon of the long palmar and the tendon of long flexor of the wrist, image 8.

Using the left index finger and thumb I lift up the skin and with the right-hand I insert the needle almost parallel to the skin. The sharp end of the needle should be pointing towards the wrist. It is obvious that you will need practice to handle this point. There is another option-technique, to insert the needle perpendicular exactly between the two tendons. With the second technique there is greater possibility for breaking small superficial veins. If the needle is inserted by mistake to a tendon then you will feel a lot of pain and you must immediately remove it. Don't be afraid, the tendon will not be damaged. It is normal if a drop of blood comes out when you remove the needle.

Another crucial point for deep stress is CV 17, dispersion. It is located at the intersection of the imaginary vertical midline of your body with the horizontal imaginary line joining the two nipples in fit men. In women you must estimate where the nipples would be if the breasts were erect as in a fit man.

The sharp end of the needle should be pointing towards the head. If blood comes out when you remove the needle, then the needle was inserted at a wrong point.

Important acupoints: Extra 1, SJ 23, Pc 6, CV 17.

Herbs: matricaria chamomilla, tilia europea, hypericum perforatum, melissa officinalis, ocimum basilicum, salvia officinalis, thymus vulgaris, leonurus cardiaca, mentha spicata, origanum majorana, valeriana officinalis, lavandula officinalis, avena sativa, verbena officinalis, achillea millefolium.

Examples of herb prescription: infusion of matricaria chamomilla or tilia europea or hypericum perforatum or melissa officinalis.

Grandma's remedies:

a. infusion of a mixture of achillea millefolium, melissa officinalis and avena sativa.

b. infusion of a mixture of tilia europea blossoms, verbena officinalis leaves and matricaria chamomilla blossoms.

c. put 5 crumbled leaves of salvia officinalis in 100ml water, drink it after 15 minutes.

Infections

During the last 24 years that I practice acupuncture I have faced numerous infections in adults and children. My daughter is 13 years and has not taken any antibiotics or other drugs.

When there is an infection, i.e. growth of microbes or viruses, we should remember that the immune system weakens probably due to stress, bad thoughts, fears, wrong diet (excessive eating, many sweet and salty), physical exhaustion (excessive labor or sex) and exposure to extreme environmental factors (cold, heat, humidity, etc.).

Acupuncture, along with your efforts to eliminate the cause, can effectively stimulate the immune system. Energy dispersion by acupuncture deprives the energy that viruses, fungi and microbes need for proliferation. The result is their easier extermination.

Important acupoints: St 36, SP 1, SP 4.

Herbs: allium sativum, hypericum perforatum, rosmarinus officinalis, thymus vulgaris, origanum vulgare, satureja thymbra, silybum marianum, olea europea, cistus creticus, origanum dictamnus, arum maculatum, baking soda.

Example of herb prescription: infusion of rosmarinus officinalis.

Grandma's remedies:

a. apply a mixture of antibiotic powder (i.e. penicillin) with honey and olive oil.

b. apply ointment of a mixture of thymus vulgaris (common thyme) and rosmarinus officinalis (rosemary). You can add allium sativum (garlic) if you don't mind the smell.

c. on wounds and ulcers place powder of dried silybum marianum (milk thistle roots, leaves or blossoms), change it every 6 hours.

d. place hypericum perforatum (Saint John's wort) oil or ointment. In old days instead of iodine solution peasants used hypericum perforatum oil.

e. put one crumbled arum maculatum (known as wild arum) leaf in a little olive oil along with 4 drops of brandy and fry it 4 minutes. Apply it on an abscess (the herb's temperature must be tolerable). Usually an abscess is treated surgically.

General cycle for the stimulation of the immune system

The first and most important point is St 36 which is located in a hollow 1cm above the horizontal plane passing through the tibial tubercle and 5cm lateral of the tibial tubercle, image 13.

The tibial tubercle is a thick bony prominence in the vertical midline just below the knee. It is found if you slide the index finger from the center of the knee downwards on the vertical midline. Immediately below the knee (the cap of the knee) is found the bony prominence.

From this bony prominence you slide the index finger on the horizontal plane towards lateral. Ignore the first hollow that you find but the second hollow, which is located nearly 5cm (the distance is the width of your three middle fingers of the hand, usually 5cm), is point St 36.

The sharp end of the needle should be pointing towards the toes, image 13, stimulation.

An exception is made when a patient who needs immune stimulation, simultaneously suffers from venous insufficiency (varicose veins) or abdominal pain or auto-immune disorder. In these cases the needle is inserted perpendicular to the skin. Normally in these cases there is a need for dispersion and the needle should be pointing towards the abdomen, image 22. There are some acupuncturists (I partly disagree) who claim that the needle has its wisdom and functions equally well regardless of the direction.

When you remove the needle a little blood may come out, it is normal.

When I start the stimulation cycle I prefer to insert a needle in the left leg of male patients and in the right leg for women (however the opposite doesn't really matter). Usually I leave a gap day (if there is an acute disease I don't leave gap days) and the next day (3rd day) I insert a needle at the same point but on the other leg. I leave another gap day and the next day (day 5) I place the needle on the other leg at point SP 1, which is found just below the inner corner of the nail of the big toe, image 15, stimulation.

I leave a gap day and the next day (7th day) I place the needle at point SP 1 on the other leg. I leave a gap day and the next day (9th day) I place the needle at point SP 4 on the other leg.

Point SP 4 is located in a hollow on the inner surface of the foot, below the tubercle of the first metatarsal, images 15, 16. To find the hollow put your index finger at the halus valgus at the beginning of the big toe. Then slide gently your finger on the smooth inner surface of the foot just below the first metatarsal. After 2 or 3 or 4cm (it depends on how long is your first metatarsal) your finger stops because of the rough and bulky eminence of the first metatarsal, image 16. The point SP 4 is located exactly where your finger stops. The sharp end of the needle should be pointing towards the ankle. If a drop of blood comes out when you remove the needle, means that the needle has been inserted in a wrong point.

I leave a gap day and the next day (11th day) I place the needle at point SP 4 on the other leg.

When you remove the needle from SP 1 and SP 4 points, press them gently (cover) for 3 seconds.

I repeat the same cycle two more times. If there is a severe disease I repeat it continuously for three moths, then I stop for 2 weeks and if there is need I repeat the procedure.

Common Cold-Pharyngitis-Influenza

"Four days I have a sore throat, mild fever up to 38°C and they told me that my throat is bright red." In viral upper respiratory infections like the common cold (sore throat, runny or stuffy nose, sneezing, headache, low fever) and all kind of flu (high fever, sore throat, stuffy nose, muscle aches, malaise) I use St 9 bilaterally, LU 5 unilaterally, St 36 unilaterally and LI 20 bilaterally. If there is fever or headache I also use Extra 1. I don't use LI 20, if there isn't a nose problem.

In the treatment of these diseases and in all viral infections the effectiveness of classical western medicine is poor. In contrast acupuncture has impressive results, sometimes from the first session.

I will not forget the wedding day of my cousin, she had fever, sore throat, malaise and anxiety whether she would hold out at all night long during the wedding feast. I chose the following points:

1. St 9 bilaterally, which is located at the intersection of a transverse (horizontal) imaginary line passing through the larynx (Adam's apple) with the line in the groove in front of the inner-front rim of sternocleidomastoid muscle (is the muscle that protrudes when the neck is extended), image 7. The sharp end of the needle should be pointing towards the head. When you

remove the needle don't press the point and it is normal if a drop of blood comes out, dispersion.

2. LU 5 unilaterally, which is located 1cm above the center of the outer half of the elbow crease, image 9. It is located on the lateral rim of the lowest section of the head of the brachial biceps muscle. The sharp end of the needle should always be pointing towards the shoulder. When you remove the needle don't press the point, dispersion and if a drop of blood comes out that means that the needle has been placed at a wrong point.

3. LI 20 bilaterally, which is located in the groove that separates the nostrils of the nose from the cheek on the lateral lower edge of the nostril, image 6. The needle is placed perpendicular to the skin. When you remove the needle don't press the point, dispersion and it is normal if a drop of blood comes out.

4. Extra 1, dispersion, mostly for antipyretic action but also for relaxation.

The result was immediate and my cousin enjoyed her marriage ceremony and the wedding feast.

Sometimes when the nose is stuffy we feel the ears "stuffy" too. Then a useful point is SJ 17, description p. 134, image 27.

The sooner you start acupuncture in relation to the onset of symptoms, the sooner you will recover. If you often suffer from pharyngitis, tonsillitis or influenza use the general cycle for the stimulation of the immune system, p. 123.

In addition to acupuncture in influenza, pharyngitis and tonsillitis you should be doing a lot of gargling (about every hour) with freshly squeezed lemon juice or salt water (half teaspoon of salt in 1/3 cup water) or infusion of salvia officinalis.

The diet should be light and free from sweet, salty and spicy foods. I recommend warm soups with vegetables and chicken.

Do not eat sweets (anything sweetened, no matter if it has sugar or if it is a ripe fruit), especially the period of discomfort in the throat because the above act as food for the viruses which are in your throat. Avoid cold liquids and drink freshly squeezed orange juice. Be well protected from the cold and the wind especially when you are sweating. If you feel cold, do home steam bath, p. 82 and remember cupping, p. 254. Relax mentally and physically.

Important acupoints: St 9, LU 5.

Herbs: allium sativum, allium cepa, thymus vulgaris, sideritis cretica, matricaria chamomilla, salvia officinalis, fraxinus ornus, artemisia vulgaris, sambucus nigra, hordeum vulgare, baking soda, mentha spicata.

Examples of herb prescription:

a. eat a clove of allium sativum, 2 times daily.

b. infusion of thymus vulgaris.

Grandma's remedies:

a. half a glass of onion juice, 3 times daily.

b. hordeum vulgare (barley) juice, p. 142.

c. infusion of a mixture of sambucus nigra (elder or elderberry) blossoms and mentha spicata (spearmint) 3 times daily.

d. if you have chills and aches in your body put a glass of champagne with two cubes of sugar in the coffee pot, when it starts to boil remove it from the stove. When it gets cool, drink it and then do home steam bath, p. 82.

e. prepare ointment with eucalyptus leaves p. 53 and rub it on your chest 3 times daily, then avoid draughts.

f. influenza: 1st day: 1 cup water with 1/2 teaspoon of baking soda

6 times every 2 hours, 2nd day: 1 cup water with 1/2 teaspoon of baking soda 4 times every 2 hours, 3rd day: 1 cup water with 1/2 teaspoon baking soda morning and evening. Drink 1 cup water with 1/2 teaspoon of baking soda in the morning till full recovery.

g. If there is a patient with influenza at home, you need good air ventilation. To disinfect the air, place in all rooms aromatic herbs like thymus vulgaris, satureja thymbra (savory), rosmarinus officinalis, salvia officinalis (sage), origanum vulgare (oregano) and even better rub them. The combustion of the above aromatic herbs and of the resin of pine tree also cleans the atmosphere.

Tonsillitis

"I have difficulty swallowing solid foods and my throat hurts sharply. My temperature is 38.5°C but I feel it is rising."

In tonsillitis, the important point is St 9, image 7, bilaterally. I also use St 36, stimulation, LU 5, dispersion and Extra 1, for antipyretic action. Do not forget to apply the general principles of pharyngitis.

Important acupoints: St 9, St 36, LU 5.

Herbs: allium sativum, thymus vulgaris, sideritis cretica, matricaria chamomilla, salvia officinalis, sambucus nigra.

Example of herb prescription: infusion of salvia officinalis.

Grandma's remedies:

a. bake crushed linseeds and as poultice apply it on the throat.

b. coat the tonsils with honey or salt.

c. gargling with infusion of salvia officinalis (sage) or saltwater (half teaspoon of salt in 1/3 cup water) or fresh lemon juice every hour.

d. avoid cold liquids.

Rhinitis

I use LI 20 points bilaterally. In allergic rhinitis and in case of common cold I also use LU 5 point unilaterally. In patients with constant runny nose, "like running water" I apply the general cycle for the stimulation of the immune system. In case of fever or headache I use Extra 1.

Important acupoints: LI 20, LU 5.

Herbs: In allergic rhinitis : urtica dioica, silybum marianum, plantago major, matricaria chamomilla, allium sativum, euphrasia officinalis, crategus oxyacantha, melissa officinalis, ephedra sinica, glycyrrhiza glabra, petroselinum sativum, iris germanica.
In patients with constant runny nose: thymus vulgaris, sideritis cretica, hypericum perforatum, ganoderma lucidum, cistus creticus, urtica dioica.
In influenza: p. 125.

Example of herb prescription: infusion of 2 teaspoons of urtica dioica.

Grandma's remedies:

a. for nasal congestion (stuffy nose) inhale over a bowl where you have put boiled water with 20 eucalyptus crumbled leaves or half crushed onion; you must cover your eyes with a towel.

Alternatively instillate 4 drops from a solution of 1/4 teaspoon salt in half a glass of water, in each congested nostril.

b. in allergic rhinitis: in the morning before your breakfast have a teaspoon (the first two days half a teaspoon) of pollen or drink the pollen dissolved in water. Repeat the remedy for 20 days in spring and autumn and ideally before the period your symptoms usually start.

c. nosebleed: press the nostril which bleeds with your finger for 10 minutes and then place cotton impregnated with infusion of origanum vulgare or with 10 drops of lemon.

Laryngitis

"I'm a singer, probably I oversang and I am also very sad because of the divorce" she says with a hoarse voice that just sounded. "Tomorrow I must sing, help me."

I chose the following points: St 9 bilaterally, St 36 right, LU 5 right and Pc 6 left. The next day I placed the needles at the same points, but in the other leg and arm.

Thank goodness she had significantly recovered and sang. In next sessions I stimulated the immune system, p. 123 and used each relaxation acupoint, p. 119, alternately.

Important acupoints: St 9, LU 5.

Herbs: malva sylvestris, althea officinalis, thymus vulgaris, salvia officinalis, plantago major, matricaria chamomilla, allium sativum, sideritis cretica, hypericum perforatum and brassica olarecea.

Examples of herb prescription: infusion, of malva sylvestris (mallow) or althea officinalis (marsh mallow) roots, leaves and blossoms.

Grandma's remedies:

a. Gargling (about every hour) with saltwater (half a teaspoon of salt 1/3 cup water) or with infusion of salvia officinalis leaves.

b. apply poultice of 2 boiled cabbage leaves on the throat. Eat two freshly boiled cabbage leaves, 3 times daily.

Sinusitis

The most important points in the treatment of sinusitis are the local points. These points are found by pressing on the cheeks and at the area between the eyes and mouth. The most painful ones are the local acupoints.

I place needles also at LU 5 and at the points which correspond to the narrow canals that unite the sinuses with the nasal cavity. These canals should be open so as the sinuses to "breathe" and expel their secretions. These points are located 1cm above and 1cm inner from the LI 20 bilaterally; do dispersion. In next sessions I also stimulated the immune system, p. 123 and used each relaxation acupoint, p. 119, alternately.

In frontal sinusitis I use Extra 1 and Bl 2 which is located on the eyebrow about 3cm from the vertical midline (the first small hollow which is found by sliding the index finger on the eyebrow, image 6.

Important acupoints: local painful points, LU 5, sinuses canal points.

Herbs: thymus vulgaris, malva sylvestris, althea officinalis, origanum vulgare, origanum majorana, salvia officinalis, matricaria chamomilla, allium sativum, sideritis cretica, hypericum perforatum.

Instillation: only one drop of ecballium elaterium or carrot or lemon in each nostril.

Inhalation: eucalyptus globulus, matricaria chamomilla, lavandula officinalis.

Examples of herb prescription: infusion of malva sylvestris or althea officinalis roots, leaves and blossoms.

Grandma's remedies:

a. in the morning instillate a drop of carrot juice in each nostril and at night a drop of lemon juice.

b. in the morning instillate 3 drops of olive oil in each nostril (if both sinuses are suffering), then instillate only one drop ecballium elaterium in each nostril (if both sinuses are suffering) and inhale. You will probably have a runny nose till night (do not lie down until it stops) and you will feel a burning sensation in the throat. Instillation of Ecballium elaterium can be repeated after 10 days.

c. inhalation therapy: breathe directly over a pot (removed from the stove) containing 1/2 L boiling water and 20 eucalyptus crumbled leaves or 6 teaspoons matricaria chamomilla blossoms or 10 lavandula officinalis blossoms or mixture of 15g origanum vulgare, 15g origanum majorana and 20 wild rosa canina leaves or a mixture of two lemon's juice, 1 teaspoon salt, 1/4 teaspoon pepper and 10 lavandula officinalis blossoms. Your eyes must be well covered, e.g. with a towel.

d. 6-day fruit therapy (e.g. orange).

Bronchitis

In bronchitis and in respiratory infection (cough, coughing up sputum and often fever) the main acupuncture point is LU 5, dispersion. I also apply the general cycle for the stimulation of the immune system, p. 123. In case of fever I also use Extra 1.

If the physician diagnoses tracheobronchitis you can additionally place needles in the sternum area at the points which are more painful when pressed.

In case of localized respiratory infection you must ask the physician to mark the skin area above the infection. Press the area with your fingers and place needles at the most painful points. Insert all the needles perpendicularly and when you remove them don't press the points, dispersion. It is normal if a drop of blood comes out.

If you fear of not taking antibiotics, then remember that acupuncture can be done while on medication.

When you suffer from respiratory infection, you must be well protected from cold, drink a lot of water or tea, eat warm soups and have a light diet free from sugar and salt. Remember cupping, p. 254 and home steam bath, p. 82.

Important acupoints: LU 5, St 36, CV 17.

Herbs: thymus vulgaris, tussilago farfara, salvia officinalis, matricaria chamomilla, allium sativum, sideritis cretica, hypericum perforatum, verbena officinalis, althea officinalis, eucalyptus globulus, mentha pulegium, origanum vulgare, marrubium vulgare, hordeum vulgare, pulmonaria officinalis, foeniculum vulgare, tilia europea, sambucus nigra, verbascum thapsus, cistus creticus, olea europea.

Examples of herb prescription:

a. infusion of thymus vulgaris, you can sweeten it with a little honey.

b. infusion of tussilago farfara, 20g in 1 L water.

Grandma's remedies:

a. infusion of almond tree blossoms before meals, 4 times daily.

b. in a blender or juicer put 10 spring onions. Strain and drink half teaspoon of the juice every 2 hours.

Otitis

The treatment of otitis externa (ear pain worsened by pressing on the tragus or by pulling the lobule of the ear) and otitis media (the eustachian tube and the nose are often blocked, pulling the lobule of the ear does not worsen the pain) with acupuncture has immediate and very good results.

I use:

SI 19 which is located at the center of the skin flap (tragus) which is shifted when our index finger is put in our ear canal, image 27, dispersion and

SJ 17 which is located behind the lobule of the ear between the condyle of the mandible and the mastoid process in a hollow that becomes larger when we open our mouth, image 27, dispersion.

The needles at these two points should be inserted perpendicularly. It is normal if a drop of blood comes out.

The first goal in otitis media is to breath free from a decongested nose, so apart from the two above points I place needles at LI 20 bilaterally. Finally, I follow the general cycle for the stimulation of the immune system, p. 123, especially with recurring ear infections.

In otitis media wide chewing movements and Valsava test (we puff out the cheeks while we have the mouth and nose closed) are helpful. In case of congested nose the use of saline water in the nose helps.

When I was a student I once suffered from otitis media with severe pain in the right ear which kept me immobilized in bed having a convenient left lateral position. The recommendation of the otolaryngologist was to get antibiotics otherwise the tympanic membrane would break and there would be need for corrective surgery. At that time I was not aware of acupuncture but I didn't like medicines. I fasted (only water) for 3 days, I ate only orange juice for 4 days and for another 2 days I ate fruit, vegetables and nuts. Following this diet therapy I fully recovered. I note that in young children suffering from otitis media sometimes the tympanic membrane breaks, fluid runs from the ear, the children are relieved and then there is not need for tympanoplasty.

Important acupoints: SI 19, SJ 17.

Herbs: hypericum perforatum, allium sativum, thymus vulgaris, satureja thymbra, rosmarinus officinalis, allium cepa, salvia officinalis.

Example of herb prescription: infusion of hypericum perforatum.

Grandma's remedies:

a. if the tympanic membrane is not ruptured and you have not otorrhea or otorragia, instillate in the ear canal drops of (depending on the muscle test for selecting food-substances) onion juice or origanum majorana (oregano) juice or olive oil with verbascum thapsus or chamomile or melissa officinalis (melissa) or allium sativum (garlic) or just tolerably hot olive oil.

b. instillate 5 drops of warm melted onion (tolerable in our skin temperature).

Conjunctivitis

In conjunctivitis (red eye burning or tingling) of microbial aetiology, the main points are around the eye orbit: SJ 23, Bl 2 and Gb 1 located 1cm laterally of the lateral wall of the eye orbit, image 6.

Insert all the above needles perpendicularly. When you remove them you shouldn't press the points, dispersion. It is normal if a drop of blood comes out.

In conjunctivitis of allergic aetiology, usually both eyes are affected, the additional points are LU 5, St 36 and SP 4.

Do not rub your eyes (to avoid transmission of microbes to the healthy eye) and blink your eyes often to create tears.

If the problem is the constant tearing, follow the general cycle for the stimulation of the immune system, p. 123.

Important acupoints: SJ 23, Bl 2.

Herbs: choose from bactericidal herbs, p. 57.

Examples of herb prescription:

a. wash with lukewarm infusion of matricaria chamomilla

b. instillate 3 drops lukewarm infusion of calendula officinalis or malva sylvestris or chelidonium majus or hydrastis canadensis. With the above you can impregnate cotton and put it over the closed eyelids.

Grandma's remedies:

a. dissolve 1/4 teaspoon of baking soda in half a glass of lukewarm water and instillate 3 drops.

b. boil a biological lettuce (lactuca sativa) in 1/2 L water. Strain the liquid and use it lukewarm for washing the eyes.

Local skin infection

Skin infection is caused from a major or minor skin trauma which allows the entrance of microbes and leads to skin inflammation (red, hot and painful skin). In case of local skin infection place needles in the peripheral limits of the skin inflammation area. Better place the needles on the healthy peripheral skin rather than on the red inflamed skin.

If the inflammation is small in size (e.g. like 1 cent euro coin), one needle is enough, if it is larger, then place peripherally crosswise 4 or more needles accordingly.

Insert all the above needles perpendicularly. When you remove them you shouldn't press the points, dispersion. If a drop of blood comes out it is considered normal.

It is also wise to place a needle at the remote acupuncture point which corresponds to the inflammation area and is located half a centimeter below the bottom corners of the fingernails or toenails, images 11, 12, 17, 18, 19 and 20. Maybe two or more remote points correspond to the inflammation area.

These points are a little painful, but are very effective. Insert the needles perpendicularly. When you remove the needles press gently for 3 seconds, stimulation. If a drop of blood comes out it is normal.

Image 11:

Point 1 is LU 11 and is located at the lateral bottom corner of the nail of the thumb.

Point 3 is SI 1 and is located at the medial bottom corner of the nail of the little finger.

Point 4 is the LI 1 and is located at the lateral (towards the thumb) bottom corner of the nail of the index finger.

Point 5 is SJ 1 and is located at the medial lower corner of the nail of the ring finger.

Image 12:

Point 1 is LU 11 and is located at the lateral bottom corner of the nail of the thumb.

Point 2 is Pc 9 and is located at the lateral (towards the thumb) bottom corner of the nail of the middle finger.

Point 3 is SI 1 and is located at the medial bottom corner of the nail of the little finger.

image 17:

Point 12 is SP 1 and is located at the medial bottom corner of the nail of the big toe.

Point 10 is Liv 1 and is located at the lateral bottom corner (towards the little finger) of the nail of the big toe.

Kd 1 corresponds to strip 11, and is located at the hollow where the red prominence of the sole becomes less red and the arch of the sole begins, image 20 and video.

image 18:

Point 9 is Bl 67 and is located at the lateral bottom corner of the nail of the little finger.

Point 8 is Gb 44 and is located at the lateral bottom corner of the nail of the fourth finger.

The remote acupuncture point corresponding to strip 11 is point Kd 1 and is shown in image 20.

image 19:

Point 10 is Liv 1 and is located at the lateral bottom corner (towards the little finger) of the nail of the big toe.

Point 7 is St 45, which is located at the lateral (towards the little finger) bottom corner of the nail of the second finger.

Point 8 is Gb 44 and is located at the lateral bottom corner of the nail of the fourth finger.

Point 9 is Bl 67 and is located at the lateral bottom corner of the nail of the little finger.

Important acupoints: local peripheral points and accordingly LU 11, LI 1, Pc 9, SJ 1, SI 1, SP 1, Liv 1, St 45, Gb 44, Bl 67, Kd 1.

Herbs: choose from bactericidal herbs, p. 57. Drink infusion or decoction in case of significant skin infection, if it is a simple one, apply an ointment of the above herbs.

Example of herb prescription: infusion of rosmarinus officinalis, you may add a little honey.

Grandma's remedy: put a teaspoon of chamomile in a glass of water. Boil it for 3 minutes, then mix it well with 1 teaspoon of baking soda and rinse the skin off. When the skin becomes dry, apply ointment made of honey, Ceylon cinnamon and baking soda in equal amounts (http://giatrosofia -bartzokas.blogspot.gr/).

Urinary tract infection, prostatitis

A woman who has painful urination, frequent urination or urge to urinate (or both) with little urine and a burning sensation during urination probably suffers from urinary tract infection also known as acute cystitis or bladder infection.

This is confirmed by urinalysis, where white blood cells (leukocytes) are present. At the same time give the microbiology laboratory urine to be cultured so as after 2 days to learn the type of microbe and the antibiotic sensitivity.

If for some reason the patient doesn't want to take antibiotics, then the best alternative is acupuncture with diet therapy. Avoid eating solid food for about three days, drink only liquids (water, herbal teas and natural fruit juices without sugar or honey or other sweeteners). If the patient wants to take antibiotics and also wants the annoying symptoms to end as soon as possible, then the patient should complementary apply acupuncture and follow diet therapy.

The most frequent victims of urinary infection are women who have sexual intercourses. Due to differences in anatomy in women (shorter urethra: 4cm, compared to 15cm in men), the microbes more easily reach the bladder, where find food (the stagnant urine) and multiply. For this reason, women should urinate before sexual intercourse so as to have an empty bladder. After sexual intercourse they should drink enough water to urinate again. The microbes are drifted with the urine before they multiply. Basic hygiene rules are necessary to be followed so as the microbes from the anus not be transferred to the urethra. Women after sexual intercourse should rest and not get tired.

We should not ignore the fact that sexual intercourse means energy exchange and energy loss. The lost energy was destinated for the creation of a new life. The energy exchange between woman and man makes the sexual intercourse so desirable.

In males the urinary tract infection is associated with prostatic hypertrophy, disruption in the flow of urine, prolonged existence of catheter, poor personal hygiene or unnatural sexual intercourse.

Prevention is the major goal but if urinary tract infection happens, then acupuncture is helpful.

The treatment in both sex is about the same.

The main acupuncture point on urinary infection and prostatitis is Bl 57, located between the two heads of the calf, image 14.

To find the point place the patient prone (face down) and slide your index finger from the Achilles tendon upwards (always in the midline towards the back of the knee). Between the two muscle masses of the two heads of the calf (approximately in the center of the calf) is a hollow, point BI 57. The sharp end of the needle should be pointing towards the knee. When you remove the needle don't press the point, dispersion and it is normal if a drop of blood comes out.

Optional points on urinary infection are local points at the area of the bladder (just above the pudenda, exactly above the hairy pubic area). In a simple urinary infection at a generally healthy female who follows the general principles of the treatment, point BI 57 is enough. Don't insert needles in more than 3 local points. Choose the local points by pressing the area just above the hairy pubic line. Insert needles into the three more painful points. Insert the needles perpendicularly. When you remove the needles don't press the points, dispersion and it is normal if a drop of blood comes out.

In prostatitis and in prostatic hypertrophy, apart from BI 57, insert a needle at a local point located 1cm above the center of the root of the penis, image 8. The sharp end of the needle should be pointing towards the abdomen and **never** pierce the skin of the penis. When you remove the needle don't press the point, dispersion.

In case of prolonged catheter, the patient needs to change the catheter aseptically and drink plenty of fluids so as to have plenty of urine. The urine color must be similar to the transparent color of the water (sometimes this is impossible because several drugs color the urine).

In recurrent urinary tract infection and chronic prostatitis without anatomy problem of the urinary tract, the urologists don't have other solution than prolonged antibiotic therapy. Acupuncture with diet therapy (fasting or fruit therapy for at least two weeks), keeping the previous rules of sexual intercourse and aseptic catheter change are the alternative solutions.

Important acupoint: Bl 57.

Herbs: hordeum vulgare, petroselinum sativum, apium graveolens, rubus fruticosus, parietaria diffusa, arbutus officinalis, arctostaphylos uva ursi, cranberry-vaccinium macrocarpon, blueberry-vaccinium vitis idaea, taraxacum officinalis, agropyron repens, cistus creticus, hypericum perforatum, achillea millefolium, equisetum arvense.

Example of herb prescription: in 5 L of water boil 1kg barley (hordeum vulgare). When barley begins to peel, stop boiling. Strain and drink a glass of it, 3 times daily before meals. To maintain the liquid, refrigerate it and when you want to drink it, warm it up.

Grandma's remedies:

a. in 1 L water boil 20g parietaria diffusa leaves and blossoms, when the water gets the color of brandy, strain it and drink a glass of it, 3 times daily (elder Gabriel, Kafsokalyvia, Mount Athos, Hellas).

b. in the first warning sign of cystitis drink a glass of water with a teaspoon baking soda well dissolved, every day until symptoms subside.

c. in the first warning sign of cystitis drink a glass of water with 2 tablespoons Ceylon cinnamon powder and half a teaspoon of honey well dissolved. The next day start eating 1 teaspoon Ceylon cinnamon powder and 1/3 teaspoon of honey, once a day, until symptoms subside.

d. in case of persistent urinary infection or chronic prostatitis: hydrogen peroxide, p. 156.

Vaginitis

Antibiotics often affect the vagina flora and fungi multiply. Other causes of vaginitis are poor hygiene and minor injuries during sexual intercourse. If vagina is not wet before the entrance of penis, minor injuries occur. When women get old or are on medication, vagina becomes dry (atrophy of the mucosa).

The main acupuncture point is Kd 10, image 14, located 3cm above the transverse midline of the knee and medial (towards the vertical midline that imaginary is between the two legs) of the medial tendon of the posterior biceps muscle, bordering with it. This point is painful when pressed. The sharp end of the needle should be pointing towards the abdomen. When you remove the needle don't press the point, dispersion. If blood comes out, it means that the needle wasn't placed at the right point.

Secondary point is St 36, dispersion, insert the needle perpendicularly. In case of mild symptoms use St 36 after the second session.

In case of recurrent vaginitis use the general cycle for the stimulation of the immune system, p. 123.

Important acupoint: Kd 10.

Herbs: matricaria chamomilla, salvia officinalis, rosmarinus officinalis, thymus vulgaris, origanum vulgare, hypericum perforatum, allium sativum.

Examples of herb prescription:

a. infusion of rosmarinus officinalis.

b. intravaginal washing with lukewarm infusion of matricaria chamomilla or salvia officinalis or rosmarinus officinalis or thymus vulgaris or origanum vulgare. In the acute phase have two washes, then one wash until symptoms disappear.

Grandma's remedy: in the bathtub, filled with warm water, pour 4 glasses of apple cider vinegar. The woman opens her legs so that the water enters the vagina. She remains in the bath for at least 15 minutes.

Gastroenteritis

"Last night I went out for dinner, I ate a lot and I mixed many different foods, maybe the pork was not so good, leaving the tavern, perhaps I got cold. The truth is that I had a very bad night, I had pain in the abdomen, diarrhea and I vomited twice."

In case of abdominal pain, the insertion of a needle at point St 36, dispersion, image 22, helps significantly, sometimes dramatically. Apart from this point you can place needles at the most painful parts of the abdomen, not more than four.

Vomiting and diarrhea help us detoxify, kicking out of the body viruses, bacteria and toxin products of poor digested food.

When you are suffering from gastroenteritis do not eat any solid food. When symptoms are intense, only water is recommended. When patient wants something to eat, freshly squeezed juice from fruit or herbal tea (chamomile) or light soup from vegetables are recommended.

If diarrhea is the major problem, then SP 4 should be the main acupuncture point. Insert the needle perpendicularly, dispersion, also use St 36, dispersion.

Antiemetic point is Pc 6, stimulation, also use St 36, dispersion.

In repeated gastroenteritis check water quality, proper food maintenance, food quality and consult a physician.

Important acupoints: St 36, SP 4.

Herbs: origanum vulgare, matricaria chamomilla, satureja thymbra, hypericum perforatum, cistus creticus, salvia officinalis, apple, ceratonia siliqua, plantago major, pistacia lentiscus, morus nigra, arctium lappa, castanea sativa, erica manipuliflora, foeniculum vulgare.

Example of herb prescription: infusion of origanum vulgare, 1-3 times daily.

Grandma's remedies:

a. eat a mixture of 7 drops of lemon juice and a teaspoon of raw Hellenic coffee powder, only once.

b. drink 30ml of vinegar, only once (http://giatrosofia -bartzokas. blogspot.gr/).

c. drink a juice of half a lemon, only once.

Herpes Zoster

If you haven't experienced pain, you can't understand patients suffering from herpes zoster. One of the worst pains is herpes zoster pain. Acupuncture is an effective therapy for this viral disease.

I use point St 36, stimulation and a point in the spine, dispersion. The spine point is located in the midline at the same horizontal level of the rash (the target is the infected spinal ganglia). You can also insert needles (no more than four) in the most painful points. Insert the needles beside the rash, always in the nearby unaffected skin.

You should follow the general cycle for the stimulation of the immune system, p. 123. Insert needles every day, until the intense symptoms subside.

In case of rash on the lips insert a needle in the unaffected nearby skin (not in the lip mucosa), dispersion. You should also follow the general cycle for the stimulation of the immune system, p. 123. Apply white spirit or alcohol on the lip rash many times every day.

In both cases don't forget that the immune system weakens due to stress, constant thoughts, fear, wrong diet (excessive eating, sweet and salty food), physical exhaustion (excessive labor or sex) and exposure to extreme environmental factors (cold, heat, humidity, etc.).

Use relaxation acupuncture points, watch your diet and take charge of your life.

Important acupoints: St 36, spine point.

Herbs: hypericum perforatum, melissa officinalis, thymus vulgaris, rosmarinus officinalis, cistus creticus, salvia officinalis, glycyrrhiza glabra, astragalus spruneri, mentha piperata, plantago major, viola tricolor.

Example of herb prescription: infusion of hypericum perforatum.

Grandma's remedies:

a. apply ointment of one of the above mentioned herbs or apply olive oil with hypericum perforatum many times every day.

b. in case of itching apply carrot juice poultice.

c. apply lemon juice, if you get irritated, apply olive oil or olive oil with hypericum perforatum.

c. hydrogen peroxide, p. 156.

Diabetes mellitus

There are two types of diabetes, type I (juvenile or insulin-dependent) and type II (adult).

In type I diabetes, which unfortunately occurs in young people with a peak age of 10 to 13 years, the b-cells of the islets of Langerhans in the pancreas, responsible for insulin production, are totally or almost totally destroyed from the auto-immune system. Using acupuncture is difficult to stop the need for insulin but you might decrease the amount of insulin.

In type II diabetes (adult type) the causes are obesity, sedentary lifestyle with lack of exercise and stress.

The chronic complications of diabetes are vascular diseases as coronary artery disease, peripheral artery disease, cerebrovascular disease, retinopathy, nephropathy, neuropathy and no vascular diseases as gastroparesis, infections and skin changes.

Follow the general cycle for the stimulation of the immune system, p. 123 and use acupoints for relaxation, p. 119.

Knowing the causes of diabetes we can administer treatment. First of all we decrease the amount of food and we avoid sweets and any sweet food. When a food doesn't contain sugar, it may contain other sweeteners (sometimes worse than sugar). Diabetics must avoid every sweet food, even pure honey or fresh sweet fruit as banana or melon. Chew food very well, especially starchy food (bread, pasta, potatoes, rice). The key is to eat less and mainly pure organic foods. Obesity is the number one cause of diabetes.

By exercising not only do we lose weight, but we improve the functioning of the entire body and we increase the consumption of blood glucose as well. That is why regular exercise is essential for diabetics. Walking in nature also offers relaxation. Leave your house and go tracking.

Herb therapy is very helpful.

Do not forget to check regularly the glycosylated hemoglobin (blood test) to determine whether the mean value of glucose is in normal range.

Important acupoints: St 36, CV 17.

Herbs: allium cepa, rubus fruticosus, cinnamomum zeylanicum, taraxacum officinalis, cichorium intibus, viscum album, blueberry-vaccinium vitis idaea, urtica dioica, equisetum arvense, rubus fruticosus, cistus creticus, cucumber, origanum majorana, carrot, thymus vulgaris, salvia officinalis, allium sativum, tragopogon porrifolius, allium porrum, avena sativa, plantago major, ceratonia siliqua, olea europea, almond tree, quercus coccifera, ginseng, sarcopoterium spinosum, cupressus sempervirens, mercurialis annua, pinus halepensis, hypericum perforatum, achillea millefolium, aloe vera, brassica olarecea, apple, lemon, petroselinum sativum.

Examples of herb prescription:

a. infusion of rubus fruticosus (12 crumbled leaves in a glass of water).

b. boil 100 small leaves (20g) olea europea in 1 L water for 15 minutes, drink 100ml, 3 times daily.

c. drink 30ml raw onion juice before breakfast, daily.

d. drink one teaspoon of tincture of allium sativum before breakfast, daily. To make this tincture, put 3 crushed onions in 1 L rakee for 2 weeks, keep it in a dark place.

e. drink a glass of carrot juice, 2 times daily.

Grandma's remedies:

a. cut a root of quercus coccifera (preferably growing over 700m) into very small pieces. Boil 650g of the root in 2 L water for 2-3 hours, in low temperature until 500ml water remains. Take it out of the stove and add 150ml 95 degrees pure alcohol. Place it in the refrigerator (for indefinite maintenance) and drink 30ml immediately after the meal, 3 times daily. Treatment lasts for 20 days without a need for a restricted diet (monk Pachomios Tsakonas). Yet do not eat a lot of sweets or sweetened foods.

b. eat bitter almonds as follows: in the morning before having breakfast eat one bitter almond, the next morning 2, the third morning 3, the fourth 4, the fifth 5, the sixth 6, the seventh 7, the eighth eat 6 bitter almonds, the ninth 5, the tenth 4, the eleventh 3, the twelfth 2 and the thirteenth eat one bitter almond and stop. If you find that it is beneficial, repeat it after 1 month.

c. boil the peels from 5 lemons in 1.2 L water till 300ml remains. Drink 60ml, 1-3 times daily.

d. hydrogen peroxide, p. 156.

e. fasting, fruit therapy and raw food diet help.

AIDS

Acupuncture can be applied in acquired immune deficiency syndrome, known as AIDS, independently or simultaneously with conventional medicine. It is beneficial to asymptomatic and symptomatic patients.

If you are suffering from AIDS you should realize that in order to improve your immune system you must change your way of life.

Empty your mind of thoughts, pray, have faith, relieve your soul going to a sincere confession, forget TV, step outside, walk in gardens, parks, forests, feed animals, do charity, sleep early in the evening and wake up cheerful in the morning full of energy.

Follow the relaxation techniques which I analyze in the first chapter.

Exercise every day, take advantage of thermal baths and herbs.

Follow the Mediterranean diet by eating less and only pure organic foods without sweet, salty, spicy or processed industrial foods.

Fasting or eating only fruit, or eating vegetables, fruit and non processed nuts for a specific period could be a weapon against AIDS.

Finally we must never forget Divine Providence, leave our lives in His hands.

The above advice on the way of life should be applied to any serious disease.

Follow the general cycle for the stimulation of the immune system, p. 123 and every day use one relaxation acupoint, p. 119.

Important acupoints: St 36, CV 17.

Herbs: allium sativum, hypericum perforatum, origanum vulgare, thymus vulgaris, allium cepa, sambucus nigra, hyssopus officinalis, arctium lappa, aloe vera, glycyrrhiza glabra, cistus creticus, echinacea angustifolia, viscum album.

Example of herb prescription: garlic therapy, p. 63.

Grandma's remedies:

a. hydrogen peroxide, p. 156.

b. try not to think the same thing twice a day!

Cancer

Should we tell the patient that has malignant brain tumor and has two months of life remaining or should we speak for a simple cyst that needs to be removed (surgery) or radiated or treated by medications (chemotherapy)?

A monk gave me the answer to this question. If the patient is spiritually ready, then there is no need to tell him the truth. If the patient is spiritually unprepared, we should tell him the truth in order to be prepared by confession, penance, Holy Communion or any other request made by his spiritual guide.

Many priests and spiritual people believe that cancer is a blessing because God informs us that our life on earth ends, so He gives us a chance to prepare ourselves for eternal life.

Saint Paisios said that in the last years of his life he was spiritually benefited more from cancer than his intense efforts to reach God before his illness. He also said that cancer is sorrow.

The physician Dr. Ryke Geerd Hamer, who was imprisoned for his ideas, succeeded very high rates of 5-year survival in patients with advanced cancer. He believes that specific emotional conflicts and psychic shocks are the causes of cancer in particular organs:

Adrenal cortex-Wrong direction, gone astray

Bladder-Ugly conflict, dirty tricks

Bone-Lack of self-worth, inferiority feeling

Breast milk gland-Involving care or disharmony

Breast milk duct-Separation conflict

Breast, left (right-handed)-Conflict concerning child, home, mother

Breast, right (right-handed)-Conflict with partner or others

Bronchials-Territorial conflict

Cervix-Severe frustration

Colon-Ugly indigestible conflict

Esophagus-Cannot have it or swallow it

Gall Bladder-Rivalry conflict

Heart-Perpetual conflict

Intestines-Indigestible chunk of anger

Kidneys-Not wanting to live, water or fluid conflict

Larynx-Conflict of fear and fright

Liver-Fear of starvation

Lung-Fear of dying or suffocation, including fear for someone else

Lymph glands-Loss of self-worth associated with the location

Melanoma-feeling dirty, soiled, defiled

Middle ear-Not being able to get some vital information

Mouth-Cannot chew or hold it

Pancreas-Anxiety-anger conflict with family members, inheritance

Prostate-Ugly conflict with sexual connections or connotations

Rectum-Fear of being useless

Skin-Loss of integrity

Spleen-Shock of being physically or emotionally wounded

Stomach-Indigestible anger, swallowed too much

Testes and Ovaries-Loss conflict

Thyroid-Feeling powerless

Uterus-Sexual conflict

The conflicts for some other diseases are as follows:

Diabetes and hypoglycemia: A right-handed female develops hypoglycemia from anxiety and revulsion, if left-handed she develops insulin-dependent diabetes. A right-handed male develops insulin-diabetes from a conflict of resisting or struggling against something, if left-handed he develops hypoglycemia.

Heart infarct: fight for territory or its content.

Hemorrhoids: both, a right-handed woman with an identity

conflict and also a left-handed man with territorial anger in the healing phase will get hemorrhoids.

Multiple sclerosis and Paralysis: inability to escape or continue on or to hold on to or not knowing what to do.

Facial paralysis: fear of losing face, having been made a laughing stock.

Psoriasis involves separation conflict concerning mother, father, family, home, friends or pets.

Vitiligo, Leukoderma: ugly or brutal separation conflict.

Dr. Ryke Geerd Hamer first tries to find the cause of the psychic shock (which usually occurred 1-2 years before the cancer), then the patient must realize the cause and reverse it at the conscious and the subconscious level (http://www.newmedicine.ca).

Most patients when they hear the word cancer become shocked which aggravates their already fragile health. There are many forms of cancer and in many cases they are curable or the patient can live many years with a good quality of life.

Do not associate cancer with death, try to fast or eat only small amounts of pure natural foods, pray and listen to your spiritual guide. Love and faith are the most powerful forces that we have, don't waste them.

If you have the energy, walk briskly for half an hour, ideally in nature, 6 times a week; sweating detoxifies you, the rise of endorphins causes mental euphoria and the light movement of internal organs is a wonderful therapeutic massage. Try alternating brisk walking with running, then walk, then run. However, be careful never to overdo it. Work within your limits, however modest these may be. Exercise oxygenates your body properly, and, since cancer cells are anaerobic, they hate oxygen. Breathing exercises are the alternative solution if walking is impossible.

Herbs which relax and stimulate the immune system, thermal waters, proper sleep (an adult should sleep at least 6 hours during the night, the sleep from 22.00 to 04.30 is the most beneficial), hypnotism, positive thinking and the belief that real life is after death should be the weapons against cancer.

God wouldn't test us, if we couldn't bear the test and didn't improve through this test.

Cancer pathology is that cancer cells multiply much faster than normal cells and that the body immune system is unable to destroy the abnormal-cancer cells.

Acupuncture works in the following ways:

1st Cancer cells need increased amounts of energy because they proliferate much faster than normal cells. Remember that needles act as wise energy pipes between the skin (acupuncture points) and the air. Depending on where there is more energy the pipe (needle) transfers energy to the side where there is less energy. This way needles remove from cancer cells the necessary energy to be proliferated. So if there is cancer in the abdomen you should place needles locally in the skin abdomen just above the cancer area and you should also insert a needle at St 36, dispersion. Remember that fasting (eat nothing and drink only water) deprives the body energy and only healthy cells survive.

2nd After energy deprivation the next step is to stimulate the immune system to destroy cancer cells. Follow the general cycle for the stimulation of the immune system, p. 123.

3rd There are body areas where the energy has been reduced because of the disease. To increase body energy insert energy from the atmosphere through acupuncture. For example in brain cancer which causes weakness in the upper extremity you should place needles for stimulation as I describe for cerebral stroke, p. 212 and use head acupoints for dispersion.

4th Acupuncture can help you overcome the side effects of chemotherapy, radiotherapy or surgery. Side effects are treated as diseases the way I describe them in the corresponding chapters, e.g. for vomiting see gastroenteritis, p. 144.

Important acupoints: relaxation acupoints, p. 141 and depending on the cancer, e.g. in gastrointestinal: St 36, urinary: Bl 57, genital: Kd 10, lung: LU 5, brain (depends on localization): Extra 1 or SJ 23 or Bl 10, leukemia: SP 4 and breast: St 18 (p. 243, image 8).

Herbs: nearly for all herbs, vegetables and fruit anti-cancer properties have been reported. Allium sativum, arum maculatum, olea europea, hypericum perforatum, crocus sativus, artemisia vulgaris, cistus creticus, cypress leaves, apricot kernel, apple, viscum album, petroselinum sativum, apium graveolens, matricaria chamomilla, curcuma longa, ginger, olea europea, allium cepa, brassica olarecea, broccoli, mercurialis annua, quercus coccifera, crategus oxyacantha, chelidonium majus, baking soda, triticum, hordeum vulgare.

Examples of herb prescription:

a. garlic therapy, p. 63.

b. arum maculatum therapy, p. 70.

c. olea europea, p. 61.

d. boil 50g mercurialis annua leaves in 1 L water for 20 minutes, drink 1/2 glass of it, 3 times daily.

Grandma's remedies:

a. remove the thorns from 3 leaves of aloe vera (older than 3 years and without been watered for 40 days) and grind them thoroughly in a blender. Add 1/2Kg of honey and 3 tablespoons rakee. Half an hour before meals, eat a tablespoon, 3 times a day.

b. boil 1Kg barley (hordeum vulgare) in 5 L water. When barley begins to peel, turn off the stove. Strain and refrigerate it; before its use boil it a little. Before meals, drink a glass of it, 3 times daily. You may also eat the remaining barley.

c. wheatgrass juice. Plant wheat in a window box in rich soil. When green grass (shoots) reaches a height of about 15cm cut it, use cold press juicer and get the juice. Drink up to 2 tablespoons three times a day, it is said to be ideal in leukemia and generally in blood diseases.

d. diet only with water and sprouts from wheat, alfalfa, lentils, p. 36.

e. baking soda, look it up on the internet.

f. mix well 1/2 lemon juice and 1/2 teaspoon of baking soda in 350ml water, drink once daily.

g. hydrogen peroxide 35% food grade certified. Mandatory, at least 1 hour before meals or 3 hours after eating and at least 3 hours prior to sleep. It is necessarily to dissolve the drops in a cup made only of glass which contains water for injection (distilled, not deionized water); for each volume of drops add 11 volumes of water for injection, i.e. 10ml drops should be dissolved in 110ml water for injection. In other words you have to convert hydrogen peroxide 35% in hydrogen peroxide 3%. You can dissolve up to 5 drops in 150ml water for injection. Use only glass dropper.

Day	Number of drops	Times daily
1st	3	3
2nd	4	3
3rd	5	3
4th	6	3

5th	7	3
6th	8	3
7th	9	3
8th	10	3
9th	12	3
10th	14	3
11th	16	3
12th	18	3
13th	20	3
14th	22	3
15th	24	3
16th	25	3

Cancer patients continue to drink 25 drops 3 times daily for another 45 days, then they drink the same number of drops 2 times daily and gradually discontinue the therapy. The treatment can last up to six months, depending on the course of the disease.

This therapy is prohibited in patients with transplanted tissue or organ, risk of rejection.

The additional intake of vitamin E and kefir (acidophilus) may also help.

For other less serious diseases, you can find various protocols on the internet, e.g. after the 3rd day you continue with 5 drops 3 times daily depending on the severity of the disease, till the eradication of disease.

h. check the location of the bed of the patient, p. 239.

i. chanting in church or saying repeatedly: i, e, a, o, ou improve our internal organs through vibrations. Chanting i i i i i i..., we aim for the brain, with e e e e e e ... we help the neck, with a a a a a a .... we vibrate the chest, lungs, genital area and lower urinary tract, with o o o o o o ... we affect the heart and the thymus gland, with ou ou ou ou ou ou .... we vibrate the abdomen. The vibrations are transferred to and improve our whole body.

j. breathing exercises, look it up on the internet.

Low Back pain

Low back pain is one of the most common diseases which are effectively treated with acupuncture. Medication such as Nonsteroidal Anti-Inflammatory Drugs (NSAIDs) is often contraindicated with coexisting diseases such as gastritis, hypertension, impaired renal function or blood problems. Nowadays many patients, especially young people, are afraid to take medication because of the side effects. We should not forget that in older adults the most common cause of kidney failure is the Nonsteroidal Anti-Inflammatory Drugs (NSAIDs).

In other cases medication is not effective or recommended on a chronic basis, results are temporary and patients may want to avoid surgery at all costs.

Acupuncture has much better results in chronic low back pain than conventional medical treatment, as it is demonstrated by the nationwide German study.

In the case of low back pain the nerve roots are not compressed and irritated as in sciatica, but usually the cause is muscle spasm by abrupt fatigue (weightlifting), abrupt movements, anxiety or cold especially after sweating.

Low back pain when at rest or unassociated with specific postures should raise the index of suspicion for an underlying cause such as fracture, infection, spine tumor, referred pain from viscera origin. Intense low back pain at rest with sweat and raised cardiac pulses indicates rupture of aorta which needs emergency hospital treatment.

Usually the real cause of low back pain is the little, mild, moderate, or severe loss of kidney energy (do not confuse renal failure with loss of kidney energy, it is totally different). Don't you find very strange the fact that in the past older adults lifted so many weights without ever complaining for back pain and nowadays so many young people suffer from back pain, sciatica and many of them are treated with surgery? This is due to body degeneration which results from bad nutrition (overeating, plastic and unnatural food, lots of sugar, salt and artificial additives, chemical toxins in the fields), air and water pollution, radiation, anxiety to earn a lot of money to fulfill our constantly increasing consuming needs, etc. .

For low back pain, back pain, infertility, hypothyroidism, osteoporosis and dwarfism I follow the general cycle for the stimulation of the kidneys (I mean the kidney energy and not anatomical kidneys), p. 160, because there is renal energy failure.

Use local heat (heating pad, patches, lamp, blankets, etc.), homemade spa, steam bath and mild fitness exercises that relax you without causing you pain or other symptoms.

Lying down on bed is usually useful, the time duration is personalized, as long as you feel it helps you, lie in a position which relieves your pain.

Important acupoints: Gb 31, Kd 1, Kd 3, p. 160.

Herbs: cistus creticus, sideritis cretica, urtica dioica, hypericum perforatum, matricaria chamomilla, salix alba, urtica dioica, arum maculatum, origanum vulgare, trigonella foenum graecum, olea europea, achillea millefolium, plantago major), globularia alypum, ptilostemon chamaepeuce, helichrysum stoehas, astra-galus spruneri.

Example of herb prescription: infusion of cistus creticus.

Grandma's remedies:

a. in a blender blend well 2 big onions (with their peel), 1 me-dium lemon (with its peel), 10 -15 small red chili peppers, a cup (180ml) of olive oil, a cup of white alcohol, half a cup of salt, half a cup of corn flour. Keep the mixture in the refrigerator. Lay a piece of cotton on the pain area and place two tablespoons of the mixture on the cotton. Cover it with another piece of cotton, like a toast and wrap the whole area with transparent food film. You can stabilize it with a lumbar belt. Add, between the two cotton pieces, a new tablespoon from the mixture, 3-4 times daily. wear it day and night. There is no need to stay in bed, http://giatrosofia -bartzokas.blogspot.gr/.

b. lumbar massage with broth of boiled cabbage.

c. apply heat e.g. with a hair dryer and then have lumbar massage with olive oil with chamomile or hypericum or oregano, p. 53.

d. boil the peels of 2 apples in 1/2 L water. When the water be-comes half, drink it lukewarm, half an hour before meal. Repeat it for 15 days, stop for 10 days and restart.

General cycle for the stimulation of the kidneys

Initially insert the needle at Gb 31, (the left acupoint for men and the right for women), images 21 and 22, which is easy to find if you have the body at attention position (standing or lying down) with outstretched hands and fingers stuck at the side of your body. The acupuncture point is where the middle finger touches the lateral side of the thigh (it is a little pit where, if we press, there is intense pain). When we were little, we hit it with the knee and paralyzed the leg. The sharp end of the needle should be pointing towards the toes and when you pull it press the point for 3 seconds, stimulation. In the next session insert the needle at Gb 31 on the other leg.

In the third session insert the needle at Kd 1 p. 138, on the other leg, stimulation.

In the fourth session insert the needle at Kd 1 on the other leg.

Then for two more sessions (alternating left-right) insert the needle at Kd 3 located right in the groove, in the middle of the imaginary horizontal line connecting the medial malleolus (the inside of the ankle) with the Achilles tendon, image 15. The sharp end of the needle should be pointing towards the abdomen, stimulation.

The general cycle for the stimulation of the kidneys consists of six sessions and we can repeat it depending on the improvement of the symptoms.

In acute low back pain, often called "lumbago" (severe pain which won't let us bend over), we can do acupuncture every day (a session or even two when the pain is extreme). The less severe the symptoms, the more sparsely we can have the sessions (two or three per week).

The most appropriate acupoints in low back pain are remote (away from the low back).

In every session, except from the aforesaid remote points of the general cycle for the stimulation of the kidneys, we can apply acupuncture at the points of the low back which hurt (are painful), or at the points (trigger points) which are painful when pressed. If there are painful points, we are not looking for trigger points. Insert needles in the most painful points but in no more than three.

Sometimes I also use Bl 40, image 14, especially when the patient has warm footpads and is stressed. Usually it is a less effective remote acupoint. It is located at the center of the back of the knee (intersection point of the vertical midline with the horizontal midline). The sharp end of the needle should be pointing towards the abdomen, dispersion.

Back pain

"Doctor, my back is killing me; it is hard to find a place to relieve myself; only when I stand completely straight up I relax a little. I must have gotten a cold; I do have a lot in my mind as well; work won't let me get as much rest as I need; I will find some peace of mind when I rest once and for all."

Many people suffer from back pain which becomes more intense with certain movements, while it is relieved with other movements. Often back pain is constant and persists despite of physiotherapy. Patients seek warmth and massage.

The most important point is Kd 1, stimulation. You can also choose local painful points (no more than two) but usually the effect of acupuncture remains the same. Apply acupuncture for relaxation, p. 119. The results are very often impressive and superior to the ones that medications have. If you are relieved by the application of acupuncture, then you can repeat the sessions twice a week.

Relaxation, local heat (heating pad, patches, blankets etc), homemade spa and cupping therapy are helpful. Be careful of draught after local heat application. Exercise yourselves daily. Stretch your back to strengthen and relax your muscles; you can find various exercises on the internet.

Important acupoints: Kd 1, CV 17.

Herbs: same as those of low back pain, p. 158.

Example of herb prescription: infusion of tilia europea.

Grandma's remedy: boil 200g thymus vulgaris or 200g leaves inula viscosa or 500g pinus halepensis (a branch with needles) or all of them in 5 litres water for 10 minutes. Turn off the stove and leave them half an hour covered. Strain the decoction and pour it in the bathtub. There, it is good to relax for half an hour making sure that the water is at the desired temperature.

Sciatica

"Doctor, I had the carpets fitted yesterday, then I couldn't stand up straight and I still feel pain from the low back to behind the thigh and it radiates down below the knee."

Sometimes your low back hurts and at the same time you feel pain, numbness or weakness in your legs; other times your low back does not hurt but you have symptoms on one or both your legs.

Usually the nerve roots are irritated-compressed because of lumbar disc disease (protrusion or herniation of the intervertebral disk), resulting in pain, numbness, dysesthesias or even weakness of lower extremities.

Often pain is same along a strip that starts from low back area and reaches toes. In this case I insert a needle at the lowest point of the painful strip. If it is not a point but is an area, then I press the skin and I choose the two most painful points.

When a powerful acupoint is near the lowest point, then I use it.

If the painful strip is at the back side of the leg and reaches the calf, the powerful acupuncture point is Bl 57. The sharp end of the needle should be pointing towards the knee, dispersion.

If the painful strip is at the lateral side of the leg and reaches the calf, the powerful acupuncture point is the Gb 37, image 22. It is found by sliding the index finger from the lateral malleolus upwards (to the knee) on the lateral (outer) surface of the leg. It is located approximately 10cm from the lateral malleolus and it is in a hollow, between the muscles of the anterior and posterior surface of the leg. The sharp end of the needle should be pointing towards the knee, dispersion.

When the lowest area of the painful (or numb) strip is at the back side of the knee, I use Bl 40. The sharp end of the needle should be pointing towards the abdomen, dispersion.

Apart from the lowest point of leg pain, I rarely insert two needles at the lumbar level where the disorder is originated; one in the middle lumbar vertical line and the other a centimeter beside (on the side of leg pain).

When the lumbar disc disease level is L4-L5, the symptoms are usually localized at the lateral (outer) side of the leg, right down to the big toe. This level corresponds to the imaginary horizontal line connecting the upper points of the iliac crests.

When the lumbar disc disease level is L3-L4, the symptoms are usually localized at the front side of the thigh right down to the inner side of the leg. This level is 4cm above the L4-L5.

When the lumbar disc disease level is L5-S1 (located 4cm below L4-L5), the symptoms are usually localized at the back of the leg.

There is a disease called lumbar spinal stenosis in which the lumbar dural sac and the containing nerve rootlets are compressed. The spinal canal narrows due to hypertrophy of bones, ligaments and joints, as seen at lumbar CT and MRI. The symptoms are numbness and pain in the legs precipitated by walking and prolonged standing. Pain is relieved by flexion of the waist or by 5 minutes rest (intermittent neurogenic claudication). The greater the stenosis, the less distance the patient can walk without having to rest. Symptoms gradually worsen and the patients "are forced" to have surgery. Spinal stenosis surgery is usually successful but the patients suffering from this disease are over 70 years old and they also suffer from other medical problems making surgery dangerous. Acupuncture is a solution; but how can it widen the narrow spinal canal? I don't know how it is done, but I assure you it is worth trying to place needles the same way as sciatica.

Lying down on the bed is usually not as necessary as in lumbago. If you feel that it will help you, then lie down the way that suits you. The supine (on your back) position with a pillow under the knees is preferred by most patients.

Important acupoint: the lowest point of severe pain.

Herbs: same as those of low back pain, p. 158.

Examples of herb prescription: infusion of tilia europea or hypericum perforatum.

Grandma's remedies: same as those of low back pain, p. 158.

Hip Osteoarthritis

"Doctor, my hip hurts; it used to hurt only when I was walking, but now it hurts even when I sit or lie down and some nights I wake up in pain. When I stand up, my hip is stiff and it takes 10 minutes to loosen up."

Several times osteoarthritis of the hip (hip pain due to lesions in the hip joint, sometimes extending downwards) is being confused with sciatica (leg pain due to disorders of the spine).

The characteristic of osteoarthritis of the hip is that the hip hurts after coxa movements (twisting, abduction or adduction) or by distress at the upright position.

In case of intense, nocturnal or caused by distress at the up-right position pain, orthopedics usually recommend hip replacement with an artificial one.

The alternative is to have patience and acupuncture. It is worth a try because acupuncture has no side effects, it is painless and most importantly it will save you from a long and painful post-operative period. After three sessions, you will realize if acupuncture helps and you'll find the courage to continue until you have a significant improvement.

The points which I choose are the local painful points, dispersion and the corresponding points of the toes: Bl 67, Gb 44, St 45, SP 1, Liv 1 and Kd 1, images 17, 18,19 and 20, stimulation.

If pain is at the back of the hip, I use Bl 67.

If pain is at the lateral side of the hip, I use Gb 44.

If pain is anteriorly-laterally, I use St 45.

If pain is anteriorly-medially, I use SP 1 and Liv 1.

If you don't realize where the pain is, then use Kd 1.

Acupuncture has amazing results at the treatment of postoperative pain, swelling, or stiffness after a hip surgery.

Important acupoints: local painful and the corresponding toe points.

Herbs: sideritis cretica, hypericum perforatum, harpagophytum procumbens, urtica dioica, cistus creticus, matricaria chamomilla, salix alba, arum maculatum, origanum vulgare, allium sativum, olea europea, achillea millefolium, plantago major.

Example of herb prescription: sideritis cretica infusion.

Grandma's remedies:

a. massage gently the hip using rakee or white spirit. When the hip gets dry (after 2-3 minutes) apply olive oil or olive oil with hypericum perforatum or with oregano or with garlic (3 whole garlics in 1 L of olive oil), 4 times daily.

b. massage the hip using olive oil with hypericum perforatum or with oregano or with garlic.

Knee pain

Gonalgia may be caused by various causes such as knee osteoarthritis (pain of the knee similar to osteoarthritis of the hip), patellar chondropathy, lesion of anatomical elements etc. In these disorders we feel pain that increases when we are active, but gets a little better with rest.

Acupuncture has saved many patients from knee arthroplasty (knee replacement). Acupuncture should be the first treatment option for osteoarthritis of the knee as proved by the German nationwide study.

If you decide to treat gonalgia with acupuncture, you should choose the local painful points, dispersion and the corresponding toe points, stimulation, images 17, 18 and 19.

A very effective acupoint which I use is Kd 10. The sharp edge of the needle should be pointing towards the abdomen, dispersion.

Another useful point is St 35, located in the center of the lateral side of the knee, image 22. The needle should be placed perpendicularly, dispersion.

Acupuncture has amazing results at the postoperative treatment of pain, swelling and stiffness after knee surgery.

Important acupoints: Kd 10, local painful points and the corresponding toe points.

Herbs: same as those of hip osteoarthritis, p. 165.

Example of herb prescription: achillea millefolium infusion, 2 times daily.

Grandma's remedies:

a. same as those of hip osteoarthritis, p. 165.

b. put five ripe ecballium elaterium fruit with their stalk (caution if you try to cut ecballium elaterium fruit from its stalk, it pops and the containing irritating juice can harm your eyes) and 5 crushed red chilli peppers in 500ml rakee. Inside the jar with the rakee, pierce the ecballium elaterium fruit with a fork and stir well. The mixture is ready. The longer the herbs remain in the rakee, the better for the mixture. You can add rakee or ecballium elaterium or peppers depending on how strong mixture you wish. In case of knee irritation, apply olive oil with hypericum perforatum.

Ankle sprain

"Doctor, I lost my footing and twisted my ankle; it is now swollen and when I move it a little, it hurts a lot."

Acupuncture has surprisingly imminent and ultimate results, but remember that even if you instantly feel better, you need to rest-immobilize your foot for a sufficient period, then gradually load it.

I insert needles peripherally to the area that suffers (aches, is discolored and swollen), dispersion. Four needles are sufficient; the needles should be inserted in the nearby unaffected skin.

At the same time, I insert needles at the corresponding toe points 17, 18, 19 and 20, stimulation.

It's a pity that orthopedists, physiatrists and physiotherapists which deal with sports injuries don't recommend acupuncture for faster and better cure of ankle sprain and other sport injuries.

Important acupoints: local painful points and the corresponding toe points.

Herbs: plantago major, cistus creticus, hypericum perforatum, allium sativum, sideritis cretica, calendula officinalis, urtica dioica, achillea millefolium, artemisia vulgaris, rosmarinus officinalis, glycyrrhiza glabra, potentilla micrantha, arnica montana, laurus nobillis.

Examples of herb prescription: plantago major or helichrysum stoehas blossoms infusion.

Grandma's remedies:

a. in a mortar pound thoroughly 3 leaves plantago major and 2 onions and place the pulp and juice on the affected area. Fix them with bandage, leave them for 6 hours, then replace them with fresh pulp and juice. You may cover the bandage with ice, especially in case of a recent sprain.

b. apply ointment or olive oil with helichrysum stoehas or cistus creticus or calendula or hypericum perforatum or chamomille or garlic or laurel many times a day.

c. apply crushed onions.

Fracture, osteoporosis

Recovering from a bone fracture can sometimes be a painful, tiring and frustrating process. Acupuncture, herbs and relaxation accelerate fracture healing and eliminate pain. In case of osteoporosis apply the general cycle for the stimulation of the kidneys, p. 160.

Important acupoints for fracture: local painful points, the corresponding finger and CV 17.

Important acupoints for osteoporosis:Gb 31, Kd 1, Kd 3.

Herbs for fracture: sideritis cretica, equisetum arvense, urtica dioica, symphytum officinale, taraxacum officinalis, plantago major, thymus vulgaris.

Herbs for osteoporosis: sideritis cretica, equisetum arvense, urtica dioica, symphytum officinale, taraxacum officinalis, salvia officinalis, ocimum basilicum, plantago major, calendula officinalis, thymus vulgaris, mentha piperita, avena sativa.

Example of herb prescription: infusion of sideritis cretica.

Grandma's remedies for fracture: eat apium graveolens, almonds, yogurt and drink carrot juice.

Grandma's remedies for osteoporosis: boil 100g petroselinum sativum, 60g anethum graveolens and 130g apium graveolens in 1,5 L water. When the water starts boiling remove it from the stove. Cover the steamer and leave the herbs in the water for half an hour. Strain them and keep the mixture in the refrigerator. Drink a glass of it (300 ml) every day for 5 days. Stop for 10 days and repeat it over and over again.
  For osteoporosis prevention:

a. apply the general cycle for the stimulation of the kidneys, p. 160.

b. exercise regularly (walk, combine strength training exercises with weight bearing exercises).

c. lose weight if you are overweight or obese.

d. have a balanced diet (less salt and sugar)

e. quit smoking.

f. reduce alcohol and caffeine intake.

g. relax.

Neck pain

"Doctor, my neck is stiff; I can turn my head to the right, but it hurts tremendously when I turn to the left. It was probably the draught of air from the open car window; I am also a little stressed out lately."

Neck pain usually means spasm of muscles in the shoulder-neck area and it is due to stress, fatigue and cold. I recommend acupuncture at the painful local points, at the corresponding fingers and toes points and at the relaxation acupoints, p. 119.

If an area is painful, then I also use the powerful acupuncture point of that area. The powerful points of the shoulder-neck area are:

Gb 21, which is located at the upper region of the shoulder-neck area exactly where it joins the neck; the sharp end of the needle should be pointing towards the base of the neck, almost parallel to the skin, dispersion, images 23, 24.

SJ 15, which is located 3cm below and 3cm laterally of the Gb 21; the needle should be perpendicular to the skin, dispersion, images 23, 24.

When I use Gb 21, I also use the corresponding toe point Gb 44, which is marked as 8 in images 18, 19, stimulation.

When I use SJ 15, I also use the corresponding finger point SJ 1, which is marked as 5 in image 11, stimulation.

When the painful area is at the center of the neck, apart from the painful local points, I insert needles at Kd 1 and Bl 67 which is marked as 9 in images 18, 19.

Remember to use a relaxation point, too, p. 119.

Important acupoints: CV 17, local painful points and the corresponding finger or toe points.

Herbs: matricaria chamomilla, cistus creticus, hypericum perforatum, urtica dioica, allium sativum, sideritis cretica, calendula officinalis, urtica dioica, achillea millefolium, plantago major, origanum vulgare, viburnum opulus.

Example of herb prescription: matricaria chamomilla infusion.

Grandma's remedies:

a. massage gently your neck with rakee or white spirit, when it becomes dry apply plain olive oil or with hypericum perforatum or chamomille or oregano or common thyme.

b. warm your neck with a hair dryer, then massage gently using a mixture of olive oil with eucalyptus and onion.

Cervical radiculopathy

"Doctor, I feel a burning pain in my left upper extremity which is numb and weak. I have used a cervical collar, I have taken medication but I wasn't relieved. I have had a cevical MRI; a herniated disc was found and I was told I should have surgery. I am afraid, you are my last hope."

Cervical radiculopathy means that a cervical nerve root is usually compressed by a herniated disc. The symptoms are pain, numbness and weakness of the upper extremities. Often neck pain radiates on the patient's upper extremity.

Usually the upper extremity symptoms have a strip-like allocation which extends from the neck to the arm or downwards to the fingers.

I insert a needle at the lowest point of the painful strip. If it isn't a point but is an area, then I press the area and I insert needles in the two most painful points.

Optionally I recommend acupuncture of three points on the neck at the level corresponding to the symptoms. The first one is at the vertical midline of the body on the neck and the other two are within a centimeter on either side of the first point.

At the base of the neck, where the neck unites with the back side of the thorax, we can feel the acanthoid apophysis of the protruding vertebrae, where there is often a hump, image 23.

One centimeter below the hump is level C6-C7, image 24. In case of a disc hernia at this level, the C7 root is compressed and the symptoms are located at the back of the forearm right down to the middle and ring finger of the hand.

Three centimeters higher is level C5-C6, image 24. When there is a hernia at this level, then the C6 root is compressed and the symptoms are located at the lateral side of the upper extremity right down to the index finger.

Three more centimeters higher is level C4-C5, image 24. When there is a hernia at this level, then the C5 root is compressed and the symptoms are located at the lateral side of the arm.

Remember to use a relaxation acupoint, too, p. 119.

Before any surgery try acupuncture. You should first take a shot and later drop a nuclear bomb.

Before surgery, try apart from the cervical collar which most neurosurgeons recommend, the over door cervical traction system with water bag. It is inconvenient but effective, as a neurosurgeon I recommend it as the last solution.

Important acupoint: the lowest point of pain.

Herbs: urtica dioica, matricaria chamomilla, cistus creticus, hypericum perforatum, allium sativum, sideritis cretica, calendula officinalis, tilia europea, achillea millefolium, plantago major.

Example of herb prescription: infusion of 2 teaspoons urtica dioica.

Grandma's remedies:

a. same as those of neck pain, p. 171.

b. the lumbar remedy from http://giatrosofia -bartzokas.blogspot.gr/, p. 160. Apply the mixture on the neck and stabilize it with a cervical collar.

Tendonitis

Many people suffer from tendonitis (pain in the tissues surrounding a joint, the area may be red, swollen and warm) which is caused by overuse (particular motion repeated too often) or by overload (e.g. weightlifting). Tendonitis is an aseptic inflammation of the tendon (the part connecting a muscle to a bone).

The main treatment is the tendon rest which means the rest of the whole limb.

Acupuncture can help for a quick recovery. I insert needles at the most suffering (during the particular motion) local points, dispersion and at the corresponding finger/toe points, stimulation.

Usually the result is an immediate relief but beware: start using and loading the limb (tendon) gradually and driven by the lack of pain. The tendon needs sufficient rehabilitation time.

Apply the Mediterranean diet. Relaxation always helps.

Important acupoints: painful local points and the corresponding finger/toe points.

Herbs: cistus creticus, hypericum perforatum, urtica dioica, matricaria chamomilla, allium sativum, sideritis cretica, calendula officinalis, tilia europea, artemisia vulgaris, achillea millefolium, plantago major.

Example of herb prescription: cistus creticus infusion.

Grandma's remedies:

a. apply locally ointment or olive oil with the above mentioned herbs several times a day. Optionally, prior the ointment or the oil application, massage gently with white spirit or rakee.

b. blend well 2 whole onions (with the peel), 1 whole lemon and a tablespoon of cornflour. Lay out a piece of cotton on the pain area, then place on the cotton 2 tablespoons of the mixture. Cover the mixture with cotton (like toast). Wrap it with transparent food film. Add, between the two cotton pieces, a new tablespoon from the mixture, 3-4 times daily, http://giatrosofia -bartzokas.blogspot.gr/.

c. fruit therapy for 10 days.

d. thermal baths, homemade spa, steam bath.

Shoulder pain

Shoulder pain is usually caused by periarthritis at the shoulder (a type of tendonitis); when we try to reach our back or the other shoulder by moving the hand over the head or in front of the chest, there is an intense pain at the shoulder area.

The main treatment is shoulder-arm rest until symptoms subside. Shoulder-arm rest does not mean immobilization, beware of ankylosis.

I recommend acupuncture at the one most painful point of the shoulder (during your arm movement), dispersion. I also insert a needle at the corresponding finger point, stimulation.

When the shoulder hurts mainly at its center and not at a certain point, I insert a needle at the point LI 15, image 23. This point can be found by lifting the arm up to the horizontal level. The hollow which is formed laterally of the acromion (bony protrusion of the clavicle) is point LI 15. The sharp end of the needle should be pointing towards the neck, dispersion. I also insert a needle at the finger point LI 1, stimulation.

When the most painful point is in the lateral side of the shoulder I insert a needle at LI 1, stimulation.

When the most painful point is in the posterior side of the shoulder I insert a needle at SI 1, stimulation.

When the most painful point is in the lateral-posterior side of the shoulder I insert a needle at SJ 1, stimulation.

When the most painful point is in the anterior or medial-anterior side of the shoulder I insert a needle at Pc 9, stimulation.

When the pain is located at two sides insert needles at both corresponding points.

Sometimes shoulder pain is very intense and allows only a small range of motion of the arm, beyond which the arm movement is impossible and causes acute pain. This case is called frozen shoulder syndrome, which needs a long time to be cured.

Important acupoints: painful local point and the corresponding finger point.

Herbs: same as those of tendonitis, p. 174.

Example of herb prescription: cistus creticus infusion.

Grandma's remedies:

a. same as those of tendonitis, p. 174.

b. in the villages of Valtou (Arta-Hellas) traditionally they place the edge of a red-hot wire, one centimeter above the skin in the area where the patient hurts, especially above the shoulder, without touching the skin.

Carpal tunnel syndrome

Patients suffer from numbness with or without pain in the first three and a half fingers (thumb, index finger, middle finger and half the ring finger), especially after weariness. At night the symptoms become more intense and the patients wake up and shake their hand for relief. If the disease worsens, muscle atrophy happens and objects fall from their hands.

Carpal tunnel syndrome is caused by the pressure on the median nerve at the center of the wrist, in an area called carpal tunnel. During the operation, we cut the transverse ligament of the wrist (which is the anterior wall of the tunnel) and thereby the median nerve is decompressed. Postoperatively the hand must be rested for at least 10 days. If you choose the conservative treatment, you should rest your hand and do self acupuncture.

I insert a needle at the local point on the midline, 2cm below the skin fold of the wrist, image 9. The sharp end of the needle should be pointing towards the wrist, dispersion.

I also insert a needle at the finger point Pc 9, the sharp end of the needle should be pointing towards the wrist, stimulation.

It is a pity to have an operation without having tried acupuncture. The results are impressive.

Medical advice: avoid bending or extension of the wrist and weariness of the hand. Place a splint, especially at night, so as the carpal tunnel to be in a straight line (lesser median nerve compression). Put a pillow under your hand overnight, so as the wrist to be at the the heart's level.

Important acupoints: local point and Pc 6.

Herbs: hypericum perforatum, matricaria chamomilla, urtica dioica, cistus creticus, allium sativum, sideritis cretica, calendula officinalis, tilia europea, artemisia vulgaris, achillea millefolium, plantago major.

Example of herb prescription: hypericum perforatum infusion.

Grandma's remedies: apply ointment or olive oil with hypericum perforatum or chamomile.

Asthma and chronic obstructive pulmonary disease

"Doctor, my son wakes up at night suffering from dyspnea, cough and kitten-like sounds in the chest. We have spent many nights at the emergency ward of the hospital. Such a young child should not be suffering; I wish I had the problem."

Acupuncture is very effective in both allergic asthma (symptoms associated with allergic causes, usually there is a family history of allergy) and bronchial asthma (symptoms occur when patients get tired e.g. after a run) for children and adults.

The main points are two:

St 36, if you have only one needle, insert it at this point, stimulation.

LU 5, is the second most important point dispersion.

Using these two points during the asthmatic crisis symptoms will probably recede. In order to prevent future crisis follow the general cycle for the stimulation of the immune system and have acupuncture for relaxation.

With preventive acupuncture you will experience fewer crises, shorter crisis duration resulting in reduced doses of medication; finally you will probably have the desired effect: neither crises, nor medication.

In chronic obstructive pulmonary disease the acupuncture points are the same and patients receive an unexpected help; there is a chance that you will need much less oxygen or not at all.

Important acupoints: St 36, LU 5.

Herbs: thymus vulgaris, plantago major, rosmarinus officinalis, pimpinella anisum seeds tussilago farfara, ephedra sinica, asphodelus aestivus, drosera rotundifolia, sideritis cretica, origanum vulgare, tilia europea, matricaria chamomilla, quercus coccifera, ficus carica, viola odorata, tussilago farfara, trifolium pratense, lavandula officinalis, quercus coccifera, mentha spicata, valeriana officinalis.

Examples of herb prescription:

a. rosmarinus officinalis infusion 4 times daily.

b. boil 30g quercus coccifera roots in 1 L water for 15 minutes and drink 60ml, 3 times daily.

c. boil 50g ficus carica leaves in 1 L water, drink 150ml before your breakfast, every morning.

d. infusion of crushed pimpinella anisum seeds, drink a glass of it per day.

Grandma's remedies:

a. infusion of a mixture of thymus vulgaris and plantago major, drink 4 times daily.

b. smoke well dried tussilago farfara leaves or viola odorata leaves or trifolium pratense leaves or datura stramonium blossoms or leaves wrapped with cigarette paper, 3 times daily.

Allergy

It is a sunny day, you are in the countryside at the request of your children, mom has made a lot of preparations (food, clothes etc.) and just when everyone has a good time, a child is coming crying and says, "my leg is red and has blisters".

Rather than ruining your day by leaving looking for a physician, you can apply crosswise peripherally of the rash 4 needles, dispersion. If the rash area is small, like 1 cent euro coin, place only one needle.

I also insert a needle at SP 4, dispersion, the sharp end of the needle should be pointing towards the toe. If the symptoms don't recede in five minutes or the irritation continues or the rash expands, insert a needle at St 36, dispersion. If in 10 minutes the symptoms don't recede, insert a needle at LU 5. If the rash aggravates and especially if breathing problem appears then immediately go to a hospital.

If allergy is caused by food or drug, then point LU 5, dispersion, should be your first choice.

Remember that in most parts of Hellas there are needles from plants (callycotome vilosa, lemon tree, robinia pseudoacacia, wild pear tree, punica granatum, acacia farmesiana, pyracantha coccinea) offered by nature at every moment. Those who are afraid of non-sterile needles it is advisable to have a First Aid kit in the car with needles or magnet stickers. If you do not have acupuncture needles and it is an emergency, you can use the needle of a syringe.

Allergy prevention: I use only one needle twice a week at the next 8 (4 points bilaterally means 8) points: SP 4, St 36, LU 5 and SJ 5.

SP 4: the sharp end of the needle should be pointing towards the big toe, dispersion.

St 36: the sharp end of the needle should be pointing towards the abdomen, dispersion.

LU 5: the sharp end of the needle should be pointing towards the shoulder, dispersion.

SJ 5: the sharp end of the needle should be pointing towards the middle finger of the hand, dispersion.

Additionally, I insert a needle at CV 17. So, every time I insert two needles, one at the above mentioned alternating 8 points and one at CV17.

There are many children (and adults) who are allergic to dust or pollen or plants (e.g. parietaria) or insect bites or fruit fluff. If you want to avoid medication and the isolation of your children, try acupuncture. If you don't feel confident about the points, you can come to my office, to show you how to find them yourself.

Keep in mind that there are also magnet stickers if there is a fear of needles. When my daughter was little, I inserted the needles when she was asleep. Try the self-hypnosis to reverse the allergic cause. The muscle test for selecting food-substances may clarify the allergic cause.

Important acupoints: SP 4, St 36, LU 5.

Herbs: same as those of allergic rhinitis, p. 129.

Examples of herb prescription:

a. infusion of 2 teaspoon urtica dioica.

b. boil 50g silybum marianum (blossoms or leaves or stalks or roots) in 1 L water for 10 minutes, drink 100ml, 3 times daily.

Grandma's remedies:

a. hydrogen peroxide, p. 156.

b. massage your ear at point 1, image 25, for 10 minutes.

Hypertension

"Doctor I am upset; I measured the pressure and found 15 to 9.5. Should I get a pill? I heard that hypertension is a serious disease."

Apart from laboratory and imaging evaluation recommended by your physician, you should measure your blood pressure in the morning before getting out of bed, it is the most reliable measurement of pressure.

There are four important things that I recommend:

Firstly: acupuncture. Apart from relaxation acupoints, p. 119, the most important points are two:

The most important is St 36, dispersion.

The second is Gb 31, dispersion, the sharp end of the needle should be pointing towards the abdomen, opposite to the direction of the needle in images 21, 22.

Secondly: relaxation, p. 12.

Thirdly: avoid salt, control weight and glucose. You should keep in mind that almost all packaged kinds of food, as well as all pre-cooked meals have salt. If you are overweight you should gradually lose weight. Diabetes and thyroid disorders are causes of hypertension.

Fourthly: physical exercise, walking, every day a little more. Unfortunately the most faithful followers of walking are those who have suffered a heart attack, have had a surgery and "have seen the Grim Reaper with their eyes."

Important acupoints: St 36, Gb 31.

Herbs: olea europea, crategus oxyacantha, viscum album, allium sativum, allium cepa, rosmarinus officinalis, capsella bursa-pastoris, urtica dioica, portulaca oleracea, crocus sativus, apium graveolens, ruta graveolens, melissa officinalis, taraxacum officinalis, cichorium intibus, agropyron repens, mentha spicata, leonurus cardiaca, achillea millefolium, orange tree, gallium aparine, avena sativa salvia officinalis, pear tree, rubus fruticosus.

Examples of herb prescription:

a. boil 20 young leaves (4g) olea europea, in 150ml of water, for 15 minutes. Drink 3 times daily, you can add a little honey.

b. infusion of 2 teaspoons crategus oxyacantha blossoms, small leaves or fruit, 1-3 times daily.

c. one garlic clove, 2 times daily.

Grandma's remedies:

a. boil 15g leaves pistacia lentiscus, 20g leaves olea europea and 30g leaves and blossoms rosmarinus officinalis in 1/2 L water for 20 minutes. Drink a tablespoon, 3 times daily.

b. infusion of a mixture of origanum majorana and melissa officinalis.

c. put an orange peel in a glass of water for 8 hours, then drink the water.

d. place 4 medical leeches (must be unfed for a long time) bilaterally (2 + 2) just below the navel.

e. midday nap helps.

Headache
(migraine, tension headache, cervical headache)

The first thing that comes to my mind when someone complains about headache is stress. However, I ask whether he/she has ever had a CT/MRI of the brain. We always exploit the diagnostic capabilities given by western classical medicine; Patients subconsciously wonder whether there is something "wrong", so after confirming with the tests (CT/MRI) that there is nothing "wrong", they escape from the vicious cycle: pain-anxiety-more pain-more anxiety and so on.

For relaxation use one of the known points: Extra 1, SJ 23, Pc 6, CV 17.

When the pain is diffused or all over the forehead or it is associated with insomnia or excessive drinking I recommend Extra 1, dispersion.

When the pain is limited at one half of the head or at one half of the forehead I recommend SJ 23, on the same side of the head-ache, dispersion.

When the pain starts from the neck and spreads towards the head, I insert needles at the three powerful points in craniocervi-cal area: Du 16 which is located at the center of the craniocervical junction, and BI 10 points which are located 3cm bilaterally of Du 16, dispersion, image 24.

When the patient says that the headache recedes after vomit-ing, I also insert a needle at St 36, dispersion, image 22.

When the headache of a woman is associated with menstrua-tion, apart from the above mentioned point I insert a needle at Sp 4, stimulation. In next sessions I follow the general cycle for the stimulation of the immune system, p. 123.

When the pain is accompanied by runny or stuffy nose and by allergic symptoms, I also insert a needle at LU 5.

When the headache is associated with hypertension, remem-ber St 36, dispersion.

When the headache is associated with hypotension, drink flu-ids, add some salt in your diet, check your medications and insert a needle at St 36, stimulation.

When the headache is due to coffee consumption, give it up; if you need reinforcement, insert a needle at St 36, stimulation and follow the general cycle for the stimulation of the immune system, p. 123.

If the headache comes from the eyes or the teeth, you should visit your ophthalmologist or dentist respectively.

Some medications may cause headache; consult your physician. Try to use simple medications and not the expensive and trendy ones that possibly have more side effects (including headaches). However, you should know that Saint Paisios said that medica-tions close a hole and open a new one.

Zoe is 12 years old and cannot get up to go to school; has a ter-rible headache and is lying down on a bed in a dark room; she has vomited twice and has no appetite.

Her mom is upset because her little daughter is sick once again. Suddenly she remembers a "crazy" therapist who had told her that when you really sympathize someone and you are willing to share his/her problem, you will find the solution (when you really want something, the entire universe conspires to help you find the solution). As the mother recalls what the therapist had told her in detail, she decides to try it herself. She puts her hand on the neck of her daughter (at the base of the skull in particular) and prays silently and repetitively with the words: "God, help her."

"Mom, I don't know what you are doing, but I feel better; my head is relieved and I can open my eyes", Zoe exclaimed confused but also relieved. Mom still has her hand on the neck and tries to coordinate with her daughter inhaling and exhaling simultaneously with her. Seeing that she cannot manage to breathe at the same rhythm with Zoe, she says: "Zoe, in order to become better, I want you to inhale when I inhale and exhale when I exhale." While breathing, mom imagines that Zoe's pain, through her hand, comes in her and disappears in the air through the exhalation.

"Mom, you are fantastic! Let me kiss you!" said Zoe. "Thank God", says Mom.

Follow the instructions in the relaxation section: prayer, confession, etc. . If you spend too much time on the computer, do eye movements, p. 19, for every hour on the computer, do two minutes eyes movements.

Keep fit with daily physical exercise. Treat constipation.

Important acupoints: Extra 1, SJ 23, Bl 10.

Herbs: matricaria chamomilla, tilia europea, melissa officinalis, origanum majorana, hypericum perforatum, rosmarinus officinalis, passiflora incarnata, valeriana officinalis, viburnum opulus, lavandula officinalis, mentha piperata, thymus vulgaris, tanacetum vulgare, scutellaria alpina, verbena officinalis, mentha spicata, ruta graveolens.

Examples of herb prescription:

a. infusion of matricaria chamomilla or tilia europea, especially if the cold head pads relieve the patient, 4 times daily.

b. infusion of rosmarinus officinalis, especially if hot head pads relieve the patient.

c. infusion of a mixture of viburnum opulus and melissa officinalis.

Grandma's remedies:

a. chew one ruta graveolens leaf.

b. sniff 5 drops of origanum majorana leaves juice.

c. patients suffering from migraine must avoid chocolates, milk and combining wine with cheese.

d. tie the suffering area with compresses or bandannas impregnated with vinegar or lemon.

e. place a raw potato or onion slice on the suffering area, refresh it every hour.

f. for headache due to menopause drink infusion of 10g crocus sativus in 1 L water.

g. massage the suffering area using 5 drops of essential oil lavandula officinalis or mentha piperata or origanum majorana.

h. have a cold footbath, especially if you have warm feet.

i. massage the lobule of the ear ipsilateral to the pain or the dominant ear for 15 minutes.

j. put herbs that you like in your pillow.

Depression

Depression affects each person in different ways, so symptoms caused by depression vary from person to person. It can manifest itself with sleep disorder in mild cases and even with suicide in severe ones. Unfortunately it is one of the diseases of modern society, when love and the belief that our life is a spiritual preparation and a testing for the eternal life next to God, our Father, are absent.

Our soul is tortured when we do not have spiritual goals, or moral standards while our only concern is to make money so that we can consume. This disruption worsens by food full of chemicals, polluted air, excess of concrete in our cities, gene degeneration which becomes more and more increased in each generation (resulting in diseases that previously appeared at older ages and today have become a privilege of younger people as well) and by lack of exercise.

Parents should set spiritual goals to their children and not just aim at their children obtaining multiple degrees. Young children should go to Sunday school (they do a great job there and the children are taught love, eternal values, prayer and learn to socialize); we should also teach them to go to church. Children should acquire spiritual foundations in order to endure the difficulties of life. Nowadays we do not lack knowledge but wisdom and morality.

A very useful acupuncture point, especially in case of a loss of a loved person, is Pc 6, stimulation.

An additional point for the most difficult cases is SJ 5 which is located in a hollow in the middle line of the posterior side of the forearm about 5cm above the wrist, image 10. The sharp end of the needle should be pointing towards the fingers, dispersion, opposite direction from the needle in image 10.

A patient diagnosed with depression should be encouraged to exercise, to get in touch with nature (to walk on beaches, in parks, or in mountains) and work in even the simplest jobs as an assistant.

We must constantly remember that there are people who breathe with difficulty, can't walk, feel, speak or communicate. There are always far worse problems than ours and every day we must say "thank you God that we exist".

Continuous occupation with language learning, arts (e.g. painting, sewing, bee-keeping) banishes boredom and creates interests.

Important acupoints: Pc 6, SJ 5.

Herbs: hypericum perforatum, matricaria chamomilla, tilia europea, melissa officinalis, origanum majorana, rosmarinus officinalis, verbena officinalis, borago officinalis, mentha piperata, thymus vulgaris, tanacetum vulgare, scutellaria alpina, satureja thymbra, plantago major, lavandula officinalis, quince, mentha spicata, salvia officinalis, valeriana officinalis.

Example of herb prescription: infusion of hypericum perforatum.

Grandma's remedies:

a. eat walnuts, crocus sativus, sprouts, linseeds and a little bitter dark chocolate.

b. infusion of the mixture: hypericum perforatum, artemisia vulgaris and melissa officinalis.

c. infusion of a mixture of: salvia officinalis, agropyron repens, petroselinum sativum and mentha spicata.

Ulcer, gastritis, reflux, colitis, belching, heartburn, sourness

Acupuncture most often provides immediate relief and it's worth a try.

For pain in the upper abdomen (gastritis, ulcer) or lower abdomen (colitis, diverticula), I use St 36, dispersion, image 22, sometimes I also insert a needle locally in the center of the aching area.

For belching or hiccups I use St 36, stimulation, image 13.

If the digestion of food is very slow, difficult and accompanied by belching or hiccups I prefer SJ 5, stimulation, the sharp end of the needle should be pointing towards the shoulder, image 10. In next sessions I use St 36, stimulation.

For heartburn I insert a needle at Gb 31, dispersion, the sharp end of the needle should be pointing towards the abdomen. If the heartburn is located at the upper abdomen, optionally you can insert a needle perpendicularly in the local point at the center of the heartburn, dispersion.

In case of sourness which usually rises toward the neck, I use St 36, dispersion, I also insert a needle at the local skin point corresponding to the greatest upper abdomen discomfort, usually located just above the stomach.

If in colitis (pain, bloating-flatulence, diarrhea) the main symptom is flatulence, I insert a needle at St 36, stimulation and in next sessions I follow the general cycle for the stimulation of the immune system, p. 123. After a few sessions and if you feel much better, gradually start eating food with fibers that you may have had to exclude from your diet. If the main symptom is diarrhea, the important point is Sp 4, stimulation; in next sessions I follow the general cycle for the stimulation of the immune system, p. 123.

You should not neglect to use an acupoint for relaxation, p. 119.

In gastrointestinal disorders drink only juices and infusions; it is good for a short time to avoid food. In belching I recommend light and warm foods, p. 25 while in heartburn and sourness light and cold foods, p. 25.

Relaxation, p. 12, is essential.

Important acupoints: St 36, Gb 31, CV 17.

Herbs: matricaria chamomilla with baking soda, cistus creticus, hypericum perforatum, matricaria chamomilla, melissa officinalis, tilia europea, thymus vulgaris, origanum vulgare, sideritis cretica, foeniculum vulgare, allium sativum, mentha spicata, origanum majorana, asphodelus aestivus, laurus nobillis, cichorium intibus, cinnamomum zeylanicum, aloe vera, anethum graveolens.

Examples of herb prescription:

a. gastritis, ulcers, colitis, oesophagitis: 1st. matricaria chamomilla with baking soda: boil a teaspoon matricaria chamomilla in 300ml water for 3 minutes and pour it slowly into a glass where you have put a teaspoon of baking soda. Drink it warm 2 times daily, http://giatrosofia -bartzokas.blogspot.gr/. 2nd. infusion of cistus creticus or hypericum perforatum.

b. belching: infusion of thymus vulgaris or sideritis cretica.

c. heartburn: decoction of valeriana officinalis roots or infusion of valeriana officinalis leaves, drink 75ml, 1-3 times daily.

d. sourness: infusion of origanum majorana or melissa officinalis.

e. bloating-flatulence: infusion of pounded foeniculum vulgare (fennel) seeds, 1-3 times daily or infusion of origanum vulgare or eat daily anethum graveolens or all together.

f. hiccups: infusion of origanum vulgare, drink 75ml 1-3 times daily or infusion of origanum majorana.

Grandma's remedies:

a. heartburn: drink a glass of water with a teaspoon of baking soda or drink a glass of milk.

b. hiccups: put a teaspoon of sugar on your tongue and swallow it after 30 seconds

c. ulcer, gastritis, stomach pains: eat a teaspoon of honey mixed with half a teaspoon Ceylon cinnamon powder, 3 times daily or mix aloe vera gel and honey in equal quantities and eat a teaspoon, 3 times daily.

Infertility

A beautiful lady around 40 years old enters my office and says: "I can not get pregnant and I'm mentally frazzled; I have had 8 fertility treatments, I have spent thousands of euros, I have taken a lot of hormones and still nothing. What is ironic is the fact that when I was young, I got pregnant and I had an abortion. Going to church regularly gave me a fresh start in life. Now I let God drive my life. A friend of mine told me about acupuncture and I thought that I had nothing to lose. Does it hurt? Will it help me? Must I bring my husband too?"

The usual reported causes of infertility are the reduced activity of the male sperm (the man should always go and get examined, even if he thinks he is healthy), the insufficient production of eggs and the anatomical problems of women.

The real causes are stress, energy failure of the kidneys (due to degenerate genes, fear and over-consumption of sweet and salty food) and the abortions, which leave huge psychic wounds (the anatomical ones being comparatively minor) that can heal only with true repentance and confession.

Abortion is a murder no matter the age of the fetus. In 99.9% of the cases of abortions the relationship of the couple is affected sooner or later.

When young people begin their sexual life, they should be ready to take on parental responsibilities as young as they may be or as unprepared financially as they are. They should not rely on contraception. The condom might break (especially when the vagina is dry), the contraceptive pill may be forgotten and the avoidance of ejaculation into the vagina may fail.

If for some reason there is an accidental ejaculation in the vagina, then the woman should stand up and do a lot of deep seats (bending knees with a straight back) so that the seminal fluid runs outside the genitals. She should visit a gynecologist as fast as she can.

Both woman and man must have acupuncture. Use relaxation acupoints, p. 119 and follow the general cycle for the stimulation of the kidneys, p. 160.

If the imaging tests have shown that there is an anatomical problem that can not be treated by a gynecologist (e.g. blockage of fallopian tubes), then the qualified acupuncturist should also use a local acupuncture point.

Some argue that thermal baths cause relaxation, good mood and dilation of the fallopian tubes. It is said that Queen Amalia (1836-1862) visited the thermal baths of Kythnos, Cyclades, Hellas to get pregnant.

Important acupoints: Gb 31, Kd 1, Kd 3, CV 17.

Herbs: royal jelly, matricaria chamomilla, salvia officinalis, urtica dioica, tilia europea, ginseng, hypericum perforatum, petroselinum sativum, melissa officinalis, thymus vulgaris, satureja thymbra, allium sativum, sideritis cretica, origanum dictamnus, foeniculum vulgare, apium graveolens, pimpinella anisum.

Examples of herb prescription:

a. infusion of matricaria chamomilla, 4 times daily.

b. infusion of salvia officinalis for 15 days.

Grandma's remedies:

a. women should apply warm compress with decoction of salvia officinalis on the lower abdomen and lumbar area.

b. men and women should eat the food that fit them, p. 25.

Erectile dysfunction

Men's modern disease associated with stress, with vasculopathy (which is why you also need to check the coronary arteries), with lack of sexual stimulation and with medication (antidepressants, some antihypertensives, etc.).

Acupuncture can offer a solution, without medication or surgical side effects. Use one of the relaxation points, p. 119, apply the general cycle for the stimulation of the kidneys, p. 160 and use the local point at the root of the penis, p. 141. This acupuncture point is suitable for any problem that occurs on the penis (skin rash, inflammation of the glans, swelling, etc.). Avoid sweet, salty, spicy foods, alcohol, tobacco and stimulants. Relax daily.

Important acupoints: local point, Gb 31, Kd 1, Kd 3, CV 17.

Herbs: royal jelly, hypericum perforatum, rosmarinus officinalis, melissa officinalis, petroselinum sativum, sideritis cretica, satureja thymbra, allium sativum, origanum dictamnus, matricaria chamomilla, tilia europea, urtica dioica, thymus vulgaris, foeniculum vulgare, apium graveolens, ruta graveolens, pimpinella anisum, tribulus terrestis, mentha spicata, mentha piperata, globularia alypum.

Example of herb prescription: infusion of hypericum perforatum.

Grandma's remedies:

a. same as those of phobias, p. 200.
b. eat a mixture of pomegranate, egg yolk, pepper, garlic, olive oil, honey, pimpinella anisum seeds, pinus halepensis pollen (or pine cone seeds) and infusion of mentha spicata, 2 hours before intercourse.

Kidney stones (nephrolithiasis)

"Doctor I feel a severe pain radiating from the back, down the flank, and into the groin and I want to go to pee. I pee a little and my urine has strange color."

"Nephrolithiasis" is derived from the Hellenic words nephros (means kidney) and lithos (means stone) = kidney stone. The Kidney stones are also called renal calculi. Approximately 80% of kidney stones are from calcium salts (oxalates or phosphates), the rest are from uric acid or cystine.

The secret to avoid nephrolithiasis is to have enough and alkaline urine. You should drink enough water, so as urine to have a color similar to the transparent color of the water. Urine alkalinization is achieved with the Mediterranean diet, p. 47. Add a little baking soda in your diet, eat fresh oranges and drink fresh squeezed orange juices.

Insert needles till you get medical care, you will possibly be immediately relieved. The important point is Bl 57, dispersion. I also insert needles at the most painful local points in the back, flank and groin, dispersion. Remember Extra 1 or CV 17 for relaxation.

During renal or ureteric colic don't drink water or liquids and don't eat. After the colic, combine fasting with enough water and herbs to dissolve or shrink the stone and to help it pass more easily. Spend ten days to dissolve or shrink the stones. Stones less than 0.5cm usually pass automatically. Kidney stones may be the size of sand or gravel, the treatment is the same.

Important acupoints: Bl 57 and local painful points.

Herbs: asplenium ceterach, petroselinum sativum, agropyron repens, plantago major, stigmata maydis (zea mays hairs), cedrus, taraxacum officinalis, urtica dioica, viburnum opulus, valeriana officinalis, equisetum arvense, agrimonia eupatoria, mentha spicata, apium graveolens, eryngium campestre, lemon, orange.

Examples of herb prescription:

a. infusion of two teaspoons asplenium ceterach, 2 times daily for as long as needed.

b. decoction of 50g petroselinum sativum, drink a glass of it, 2 times daily for 10 days.

c. boil 50g agropyron repens root in 2 L water, until water remains half, drink 100 ml, 3 times daily.

Grandma's remedies:

a. boil 2kg petroselinum sativum (with roots, whole herb) and 250g asplenium ceterach leaves in 1kg water for 10 minutes. Drink a glass of it, 2 times daily for 10 days.

b. boil 1Kg petroselinum sativum and 300g kernels of juniperus oxycedrus nuts in 2Kg water for 15 minutes. Drink a glass of it, 2 times daily for 10 days.

c. boil 1/2kg petroselinum sativum (with or without roots), 1/2kg mentha spicata, 1/2kg apium graveolens and 300g plantago major, in 2Kg water for 15 minutes. Drink 100 ml, 3 times daily for 10 days.

d. boil 600g petroselinum sativum and 100g plantago major in 2 L water for 30 minutes. Drink a glass of it, 2 times daily for 10 days.

e. stones with size of sand: boil 40g tomato root in 2 L water until it is half, drink a glass of it, every morning for 10 days.

f. renal or ureteric colic: hot bath helps, stay as long as you like.

g. boil 1200g petroselinum sativum and 30g olibanum in 2 L water until it is half. Keep the decoction in the refrigerator. Unfed, drink 60ml every morning, then drink a tablespoon of olive oil. The longest period that you can use this remedy is 45 days. You can only use it once in 2 years. Often this remedy has a side effect: constipation. Preventively eat food with fibers and every 8 days take a laxative.

h. **prevention:**
1. replace salt with orange juice or a few drops of lemon.
2. eat an orange every morning and a radish at the end of each meal.
3. drink a glass of water with a teaspoon of baking soda, 2 times a week.

Gallstones (cholelithiasis)

"Doctor last night I suffered from pain in the stomach area, under the right ribs and spread to the right shoulder, for three hours.

Thankfully it passed so suddenly as it came. The truth is that early in the evening I ate a huge meal, full of cholesterol. Ultrasound showed gallstones, I don't want to have surgery."

Up to 80% of the gallstones are cholesterol type and associated with eating foods rich in cholesterol. The remaining stones are associated with chronic diseases or pregnancy.

If there is no immediate indication for surgery, then at the waiting time before surgery do acupuncture, watch your diet, drink herbal infusions and relax. Then do again ultrasound to see if there are still gallstones or if their size is clearly reduced.

Insert a needle at St 36, dispersion or at Gb 31, dispersion, once daily. At the same time insert a needle at CV 17. If you feel pain in your abdomen, also insert a needle perpendicularly at the center of the pain, dispersion.

Overweight patients must lose weight, reduce (not extinguish) the high cholesterol foods and reduce the variety of foods in a meal. Ten minutes before each meal eat a tablespoon olive oil (cold pressed, extra virgin) mixed well with 5 lemon drops. Drink 1 L squeezed fresh apple juice every day, eat a radish (raphanus sativus) after each meal and drink herbal infusions.

Reduce blood cholesterol, p. 246.

Important acupoints: St 36, Gb 31.

Herbs: asplenium ceterach, petroselinum sativum, agropyron repens, silybum marianum, rosmarinus officinalis, taraxacum officinalis, urtica dioica, cynara cardunculus, gentiana lutea, stigmata maydis (zea mays hairs), olea europea, agrimonia eupatoria, mentha spicata, plantago major, apium graveolens, raphanus sativus, helichrysum stoehas, linseed, orange, tangerine, pear tree.

Example of herb prescription: infusion of two teaspoons asplenium ceterach, 2 times daily.

Grandma's remedies:

a. boil 300g asplenium ceterach leaves, with 600g petroselinum sativum (leaves and roots) and 10 chick peas in 2 L of water for 20 minutes. Drink a glass of it, 2 times daily.

b. knead a sheep bile with a little chick pea flour without water. Make 12 pills and eat one every day (a. and b. by monk Gymnasios Lavriotis).

c. boil 1200g petroselinum sativum and 30g olibanum in 2 L water until it is half. Keep the decoction in the refrigerator. Unfed, drink 60ml every morning, then drink a tablespoon of olive oil. The longest period that you can use this remedy is 45 days. You can only use it once in 2 years. Often this remedy has a side effect: constipation. Preventively eat food with fibers and every 8 days take a laxative.

d. decoction of a mixture of gentiana lutea roots, silybum marianum leaves, stem and blossoms, mentha spicata leaves and blossoms and rosmarinus officinalis leaves and blossoms, drink 150ml, 2 times daily.

e. eat a tablespoon of lemon juice mixed with glycerin in equal quantities, 2 times daily.

f. decoction of pear tree leaves, 2 times daily.

g. boil 300g leaves asplenium ceterach, 50g seeds petroselinum sativum and 20 chick peas in 2 L water until it is half. Drink a glass of it, 2 times daily.

h. eat 4 radishes in total, daily (after meals).

i. eat an orange or 3 tangerines every morning.

j. fruit therapy with oranges or tangerines for 14 days.

Phobias

According to acupuncture theory about energy, fear is due to re-nal energy failure; that is why young people are energetic and fearless, while as they grow older they get energetically exhaust-ed and their fears are increased.

Follow the general cycle for the stimulation of the kidneys, p. 160 and remember relaxation points, p. 119.

For certain phobias as claustrophobia, agoraphobia, hypsofobia and fear of certain things, there is an easy treatment which often has spectacular results.

You will need a trusted person to help you, your "therapist". You will tell him/her the 5 happiest moments of your life. It is cru-cial that you recall certain moments and not generally periods of your life. If you don't have moments of happiness, recall moments that you felt nice.

The "therapist" records the moments on a paper.

Example:

1st happy moment: the moment that I was told that I passed the University entrance exams.

2nd happy moment: the moment that I embraced my girl friend years ago. I was expecting her to return from her village and I was getting worried because her bus was late.

3rd happy moment: the moment that I lied down and fell asleep, years ago. At that moment I felt such happiness (that morning I had done a charity) that I will never forget.

4th happy moment: the moment my baby said her first word.

5th happy moment: the moment during a prayer while I had a health problem. I felt an indescribably nice feeling.

The "therapist" tells the patient to have his eyes constantly closed, to relax and to imagine every scene that he describes for

10 seconds. Let us suppose that the patient is suffering from hypsofobia.

The patient is lying comfortably in a bed or is sitting comfortably in a chair and the "therapist" says: imagine the moment that you were told that you passed the University entrance exams (1st moment of happiness), and immediately the "therapist" presses gently with his index finger any one point on the hand of the patient for 10 seconds.

The patient imagines the moment of happiness (his eyes are closed), for 10 seconds. During these 10 seconds the "therapist's" index finger presses the hand point with the same force.

The "therapist" withdraws his index finger and says: now imagine you are at a balcony of the eighth floor and you are looking down and immediately the "therapist" presses gently (with the same force as before) again the same point of the hand with his index finger for 10 seconds.

When the 10 second time expires, then the "therapist" withdraws his index finger and says: now imagine the moment that your girlfriend returned from her village and you embraced her (2nd moment of happiness) and immediately the "therapist" presses gently any one point on the forearm with his index finger. The patient imagines the moment of happiness (his eyes remain closed), for 10 seconds. During these 10 seconds the "therapist's" index finger presses the point on the forearm with the same force. When the 10 second time expires, then the "therapist" withdraws his index finger and says: now imagine you are at the balcony of the eighth floor and look down and immediately the "therapist" presses gently (with the same force as before) again the same point of the forearm with his index finger for 10 seconds.

When the 10 second time expires, then the "therapist" withdraws his index finger and says: now imagine the moment that you lied down and fell asleep after the anonymous charity (3rd moment of happiness) and immediately the "therapist" presses gently any one point on the patient's hand with his index finger. The patient imagines the moment of happiness (his eyes remain closed), for 10 seconds. During these 10 seconds the "therapist's" index finger presses the point on the hand with the same force. When the 10 second time expires, then the "therapist" withdraws his index finger and says: now imagine you are at the balcony of the eighth floor and look down and immediately the "therapist" presses gently (with the same force as before) again the same point of the hand with his index finger for 10 seconds.

When the 10 second time expires, then the "therapist" withdraws his index finger and says: now imagine the moment that your baby said her first word (4th moment of happiness) and immediately the "therapist" presses gently any one point on the forearm with his index finger. The patient imagines the moment of happiness (his eyes remain closed), for 10 seconds. During these 10 seconds the "therapist's" index finger presses the point on the forearm with the same force. When the 10 second time expires, then the "therapist" withdraws his index finger and says: now imagine you are at a balcony of the eighth floor and look down and immediately the "therapist" presses gently (with the same force as before) again the same point of the forearm with his index finger for 10 seconds.

When the 10 second time expires, then the "therapist" withdraws his index finger and says: now imagine the moment that you felt an indescribably nice feeling during a prayer. (5th moment of happiness) and immediately the "therapist" presses gently any one point on the hand with his index finger. The patient imagines the moment of happiness (his eyes remain closed), for 10 seconds. During these 10 seconds the "therapist's" index finger presses the hand point with the same force. When the 10 second time expires, then the "therapist" withdraws his index finger and says: now imagine you are at the balcony of the eighth floor and look down and immediately the "therapist" presses gently (with the same force as before) again the same point of the hand with his index finger for 10 seconds.

When the 10 second time expires, then the "therapist" withdraws his index finger and says: open your eyes.

If the procedure has been done correctly, then the patient will immediately tell that he feels much better. The last times that he imagined looking down from the eighth floor down, he felt completely different and clearly much better than the first time; he either wasn't afraid of the height or he felt a little uncomfortable. If the patient's fear has improved but remains to some extent, continue with the same procedure with more happy moments.

The success of this procedure is due to the subconscious association of the pressure (touch) with the happy thought. The pressure-touch is perceived very positively and this positive feeling is transferred (the second subconscious association) to the bad thought-fear which is then converted to neutral. The result is that the bad thought doesn't cause fear or panic any more.

Be careful: before starting the procedure, ask the patient or their relatives what happens in the case of phobia. If the symptoms are so intense and serious that there is even one chance in a million to be fatal for the patient, do not attempt to do it by yourself but find a specialist.

In case of a phobia with intense symptoms but without a possibility to harm the patient's health, I tell the patient to imagine that he is watching television and on the TV (like a film) he watches himself facing the phobia (e.g. the "therapist" tells the hypsofobic to imagine that he sees himself at a balcony of the eighth floor looking down).

Important acupoints: Gb 31, Kd 1, Kd 3, CV 17.

Herbs: same as those of erectile dysfunction, p. 194.

Example of herb prescription: same as erectile dysfunction, p. 194.

Grandma's remedies: same as osteoporosis, p.169.

Smoking

Why do you pay your murderer? The cigarette is a mild drug that relaxes you at first but then you become physically and mentally addicted. Giving up smoking needs strong will.

Acupuncture will help you:

1st. not suffer from withdrawal symptoms (stress, tremor, salivation, sweating, etc.).

2nd. to relax, avoiding the need of cigarette "relaxation". This way you get distressed and your mind escapes from overeating.

3rd. it will rarely make you dislike smoking or have intolerance to tobacco.

A smoker needs to make a solid decision. Quite often "friends" and acquaintances will offer you a cigarette. Smokers keep the memory of the "pleasure" of smoking even two years after giving up smoking. You should not smoke even one cigarette because you will start smoking again.

There are very few smokers (the exception to the rule) that can control having two to three cigarettes a day.

For smoking, obesity and alcoholism, the frequency of acupuncture is as follows: daily for five days, then skip a day (on the condition that on the fifth day you do not smoke or drink anything) and insert needles again on the seventh day, on the tenth day (two days gap), on the fourteenth day (three days gap), on the twentieth day (five days gap), on the twenty-eighth day (seven days gap), on the thirty-ninth day (ten days gap), on the fifty-fifth (fifteen days gap) and on the eightieth day (thirty days gap). For obesity, the frequency of acupuncture depends on whether you follow a strict or a mild diet. In cases of a mild diet acupuncture can be much sparser.

Of course, you can have fewer sessions if you see that there is no desire for a cigarette. In tough cases of smokers, alcoholics or obese, you can have two or extremely rarely three sessions daily.

I insert needles at relaxation acupoints, p. 119 and at three points in the dominant ear. In image 25 the points 5, 6 and 7 are suitable for quitting smoking.

Acupuncture is always applied in the dominant ear; at the right one if we are right-handed and at the left one if we are left-handed. Since it is very often that right-handed people are actually oppressed left-handed, I ask the smokers to start clapping their hands. The right-handed smokers will be hitting the left hand with the right one, that is they will put the right hand over the left hand; while the real left-handed smoker will do the opposite (they will be hitting the right hand with the left one and put the left palm over the right one).

Important acupoints: points 5, 6 and 7, image 25.

Herbs: plantago major, eucalyptus globulus, thymus vulgaris, allium sativum, hypericum perforatum.

Examples of herb prescription:

a. infusion of plantago major.

b. decoction of 15g eucalyptus crumbled leaves in 1 L water, drink 75ml, 3 times a day.

Grandma's remedies:

a. chew carrot to have your mouth busy.

b. wash your teeth every time you want to smoke.

c. if you have associated the habit of coffee with smoke, give up coffee.

d. exercise yourself to get distressed.

e. tap your thighs alternately for 3 minutes while constantly saying "although I love smoking, deeply and completely I accept myself". Six times daily.

f. massage point 7, image 25, whenever you want to smoke or for 10 minutes, 5 times a day.

Obesity

Acupuncture without diet has zero value for obesity treatment. Some people believe that acupuncture can regulate and improve the metabolism but this happens after several acupuncture sessions and after having dealt with the stress of the patient. When I tell this to my patients, their answer is: "Why should I do acupuncture then? I'll get thinner with the diet anyway." The explanation is simple when you understand the cause of obesity.

We do not eat because we are really hungry but we eat to relieve our anxiety. If we do not deal with our stress, we shall be losing weight for a short period of time (under intense repression because we do not relieve the stress) and then we shall gain much more weight than what we had before our diet.

The truth is that some people, who were overweight as children, have a strong predisposition to gain weight and any disturbance of their energy situation (without necessarily having obvious health problems) causes gaining of weight.

Acupuncture, along with conscious daily relaxation and a simple way of life with fewer demands, can significantly help to fight the scourge of modern life, anxiety.

At the same time, acupuncture (with the frequency described for smoking) reduces or may entirely cut the appetite of the patient.

I use the word "patient" for the obese because we all know that obesity is a real illness which is hard to be treated and poses a direct threat to the heart, the blood vessels, the pancreas, the liver, as well as for the whole body. As a result, it is usually accompanied by diabetes, hypertension, coronary artery disease (cardiac ischemia, myocardial infarction) and increased chances of developing cancer.

Medically, to define the obese person we use the body mass index (BMI), which is the quotient of the weight in kilograms by the square of height in meters; i.e. if a man weighs 80 kg and has a height of 1.80 meters, then divide the 80 by 3.24 (resulting from the square of height, i.e. $1.80^2 = 3.24$) and the result is 24.69. The normal BMI for both men and women is 19-26. A BMI from 25 to 30 is considered overweight. A person is considered to be obese when their BMI exceeds 30.

The treatment for the obese, as well as for the overweight, has four components:

1st. Exercise, I recommend a daily walk, every day a little more; forget the elevator, park the car away from home or from your destination. Daily walking helps our lungs to function better, so that they are capable of taking in enough oxygen for the body to burn fat and eject metabolic waste products. It is also advisable to work out the joints (neck, shoulders, elbows, wrists, fingers, back, waist, hips, knees, ankles).

2nd. Diet with an aim to change eating habits, that is reduce quantity (less food), avoid salty (pre-made and preserved foods) and sweet foods, drink an adequate daily amount of water (more than 1.5 liter) and eat pure food included in the Mediterranean diet.

The diet I recommend is fasting or consumption of fruit or consumption of fruit, vegetables and dried fruit, which is intense and has quick results. Keeping an intense diet for a sufficient period of time (depending on the degree of obesity) will have great detoxifying and revitalizing effects. In cases of heavy diets it is of great importance to start regular food gradually and slowly (which has been described in detail in previous chapters).

There are also mild diets that do not affect your social obligations i.e. the diet of the half; one can eat everything, but half the usual quantity. You can fill your plate with what you intend to eat and mentally divide it in half. The right-handed should be eating the right half of the contents of the plate and the left-handed the left half. It is important to see that in your plate remained the half of the food; do not put half the portion on the plate to keep some food from being thrown away. Another mild diet is to eat nothing in the evening or eat a fruit or a traditional Hellenic yogurt (whole fat with skin).

3rd. Relaxation, there is an urgent need to train in everyday relaxation. The good thing is that several kindergarten schools teach children to exercise relaxation.

4th. Acupuncture with the frequency mentioned for smoking if one goes for an intense diet or with a frequency of two sessions a week in cases of mild diets.

Acupuncture is also applied for local fat disposal. I initially insert needles at the lower points of the areas that need slimming. After two sessions I also insert needles at the upper parts of these areas. For treating cellulite on the buttocks insert needles in the same way.

Distant points that help improve the metabolism are SJ 5, the sharp end of the needle should be pointing towards the shoulder, stimulation and St 36, stimulation. It helps to follow the general cycle for the stimulation of the immune system, p. 123.

Needles for slimming are inserted in the dominating ear (see smoking), at points 2, 3 and 6, image 25. To find the points 2 and 3 you must first find point 1, which is mentioned in the following page.

Important acupoints: points 2, 3 and 6, image 25.

Herbs: hypericum perforatum, cistus creticus, olea europea, salvia officinalis, urtica dioica, taraxacum officinalis, avena sativa, cynara cardunculus, foeniculum vulgare, allium sativum, valeriana officinalis, cinnamomum zeylanicum, plantago major, calendula officinalis, hibiscus sabdariffa.

Examples of herb prescription: infusion of hypericum perforatum or of foeniculum vulgare crushed seeds.

Grandma's remedies:

a. little garlic sauce every night.

b. eat strictly between 11.00-19.00, drink water all day.

c. tap your thighs alternately for 3 minutes while saying "although I love the food, deeply and completely I accept myself", 6 times daily.

d. massage ear point 3, image 25, for 10 minutes, 5 times daily (recommended before each meal) and every time you feel hungry.

e. drink two glasses of water whenever you feel hungry, because in reality you are thirsty and not hungry. Also drink two glasses of water before each meal so as to feel your stomach full.

f. chew food slowly so as to recognize the feeling of fullness and stop eating.

g. eat chili peppers and a few walnuts.

Alcoholism

As with other addictions (smoking, obesity, drug abuse), the fundamental problem in alcoholism is also stress. The alcoholics try to relieve their stress by drinking.

Acupuncture apart from aiding relaxation, p. 119, reduces or eliminates the withdrawal symptoms, while in a few cases causes intolerance to alcohol.

The prerequisite is the decision to stop drinking.

The needles are inserted in the dominant ear at points 2, 4 and 6, image 25.

Important acupoints: points 2, 4 and 6, image 25.

Herbs: thymus vulgaris, allium sativum, artemisia vulgaris, rubus idaeus, viola odorata, lycopodium clavatum, hypericum perforatum.

Example of herb prescription: infusion of 30g thymus vulgaris in 1 L water, 1 teaspoon every 15 minutes for the first two hours and every half hour for the remaining hours that you are awake.

Grandma's remedies:

a. put 1/2 teaspoon infusion of viola odorata in each drink (no more than 4 drinks), brings disgust, vomiting.

b. avoid spicy food-appetizers.

c. hydrogen peroxide, p. 156.

d. tap your thighs alternately for 3 minutes while saying "although I love alcohol, deeply and completely I accept myself", 6 times daily.

e. massage ear point 4, image 25, for 10 minutes, 5 times daily and every time you have drink desire.

Drugs

At the church, a woman in black clothes approached me crying and begged me to help her son. He came to my medical office, he was a strong and robust young man. He told me: "I have been heroin addict for years, but now I want to stop and I can't. My wife has also realized it, because my penis has been damaged and I no longer have an erection."

Acupuncture reduces or eliminates the withdrawal symptoms. These patients need all the help they can get. Addicted patients are in need of constant support and observation by their family. During the first week, they should not be left alone even for a second.

I use point 1, image 25, in the dominant ear and Pc 6 or CV 17 for relaxation. Point 1 is located in the center of a groove (this is why in image 25 I have placed a straight line in the center of which is the point) and when you press it with your fingernail it will hurt a lot.

It is the only case in which acupuncture can be applied up to 4 times a day during the first days. Next acupuncture sessions depend on how the patient reacts to the treatment.

Drugs must be stopped once and for all and not progressively.

Abroad some detoxifying centers collaborate with acupuncturists. In Hellas there are many drug addicts who visit Mount Athos seeking for help from the elders. Mount Athos is situated in the entire third, eastern and most beautiful peninsula of Halkidiki, called the peninsula of Athos. It is the only place in Hellas that is completely dedicated to prayer and worship of God.

Important acupuncture point: point 1.

Herbs: rubus idaeus, melissa officinalis, thymus vulgaris.

Example of herb prescription: infusion of 2 teaspoons rubus idaeus. Drink 1 teaspoon every 15 minutes for the first 2 hours and every half hour for the remaining hours that you are awake.

Grandma's remedies:

a. tap your thighs alternately while saying "although I love the certain drug, deeply and completely I accept myself", for 3 minutes, every hour.

b. massage ear point 1, image 25, for 10 minutes, every hour and every time you have drug desire.

c. seek the assistance and the constant presence of your own.

d. walk with friends in nature.

e. take up handiwork.

Cerebral stroke

"Doctor, it has been 3 months that I have been walking with the tripod, I have been dragging my left leg, my left hand has been making a slight move from the shoulder and I have been feeling very cold especially on my left hand; but I was always strong as a bull and resistant to cold. I stayed in the intensive care for three days; I was told that I'd got a stroke and was lucky to be alive.

The truth is that I always worried a lot; I smoked and ate a lot. I never watched over myself and I always took care of other people. Now I need someone to watch over me; and I was just about ready to retire and get some rest. Can you help me?"

First of all, as a medical doctor I can not foretell the future; all I can say is that I will try. The odds are in favor of some improvement (small or bigger) so I'll try to help someone who has suffered a stroke and has hemiplegia or hemiparesis. Usually the leg strengthens and walking becomes more stable; in the hand we usually have poorer results.

When only the upper extremity suffers, I apply the following set of sessions (each session is to be followed by a day without acupuncture):

In the first three sessions I insert a needle at point HE 1, which is in a groove located in the center of the armpit, image 26.

In the next three sessions I insert a needle at point Pc 6, the sharp end of the needle should be pointing towards the fingers, stimulation.

In the next three sessions I insert a needle at point Pc 9, stimulation.

In the next three sessions I insert a needle at point LI 4 located on the dorsal surface of the palm, in the corner (large hollow) formed by the extension of the imaginary lines of thumb and index finger when they are stretched and fully opened, image 10. The sharp end of the needle should be pointing towards the elbow, stimulation.

In the next three sessions I insert a needle at point SJ 1, stimulation.

In the next three sessions I insert a needle at point SJ 5, the sharp end of the needle should be pointing towards the shoulder, stimulation.

For strengthening the lower extremity at the same time with the upper (if both extremities are suffering), I apply the following set of sessions:

In the first three sessions, along with point HE 1, I insert a needle at point St 31 located at the intersection of the vertical straight line passing through the anterior superior iliac spine with the horizontal straight line going through the pubic symphysis (the base of the penis for men), image 8. The sharp end of the needle should be pointing towards the knee, stimulation.

In the next three sessions, along with point Pc 6, I insert a needle at point St 36, the sharp end of the needle should be pointing towards the toes, stimulation.

In the next three sessions, along with point Pc 9, I insert a needle at point SP 1, stimulation.

In the next three sessions, along with point LI 4, I insert a needle at SP 4, the sharp end of the needle should be pointing towards the ankle.

In the next three sessions, along with point SJ 1, I insert a needle at St 31, stimulation.

In the next three sessions, along with point SJ 5, I insert a needle at St 36, stimulation.

In the next three sessions, along with point HE 1, I insert a needle at SP 1, stimulation.

In the next three sessions, along with point Pc 6, I insert a needle at SP 4, stimulation.

I continue using again the same set of points for 3 months and if the patient is pleased, I make a break for 2 weeks and continue for 3 more months, using the same set of points.

Along with the two points on the extremities I also use one of the relaxing points Extra 1, SJ 23, CV 17, alternately.

The sooner you start acupuncture the better; if you start too late, don't despair.

Control your blood pressure according to your medical doctor consultation. Herbs and exercising will help you.

Important acupuncture points: Pc 6, St 36, SJ 23.

Herbs: crategus oxyacantha, viscum album, allium sativum, thymus vulgaris, hypericum perforatum, melissa officinalis, allium cepa, crocus sativus, gingko biloba, rosmarinus officinalis, urtica dioica, blueberry-vaccinium vitis idaea, amaranthus retroflexus, curcuma longa, matricaria chamomilla, scutellaria alpina, verbena officinalis.

Example of herb prescription: infusion of 2 teaspoons crategus oxyacantha small leaves, blossoms or fruit.

Grandma's remedies:

a. massage your weak extremities using olive oil with chamomile.

b. move or try to move constantly your weak extremities. Exercising-movement is necessary. If one little move is done, then thousands will be done.

Dyslexia

"Doctor, my child is not doing well at school; even though I help him, he omits syllables, letters (dysgraphia) and is unable to understand the texts he reads due to confusion of letters that have similar shape or phonetic affinity."

It is a modern disease that affects more and more children and parents ask for understanding by the teachers, the state and for the help of speech therapists.

Acupuncture can help these children to some extent. I use the relaxation points, p. 119, alternately. Try hypnosis or self-hypnosis.

Important acupuncture points: Pc 6, Extra 1.

Herbs: same as those of headache, p. 184.

Example of herb prescription: infusion of verbena officinalis.

Grandma's remedy: infusion of a mixture of 40% tilia europea, 40% matricaria chamomilla and 20% verbena officinalis, drink 150ml, 3 times daily.

Old age

"Doctor, my father is old; he hurts everywhere, he walks with difficulty and has begun to lose his mind. My mother also begins to age. These people have done everything for me; can I help them now that they need me?"

Older people in China insert needles every day at point St 36, the sharp end of the needle should be pointing towards the toes, stimulation; if they suffer from venous insufficiency, they insert the needle perpendicular to the skin. They do it for preventive reasons so that old age finds them able to use their bikes and be autonomous without needing the help of their relatives. They try to age with the fewest medical problems; this is achieved with daily acupuncture, with daily exercise that do every day in the squares (tai chi) and by eating less and light food.

If older people are feeling lonely or are stressed, then I use one of the relaxing points Pc 6, Extra 1, SJ 23, CV 17, alternately. I also always use the general cycles for the stimulation of the immune system, p. 123 and kidneys, p. 160.

Remember the rejuvenating thermal baths or spas. There are hotels that have at the room bathtub which provides water from hot springs, like Galini Hotel in Kamena Vourla, Fthiotida, Hellas.

Do simple physical exercises (several breaths, gentle movements of the neck, waist, etc.) and walk as much as possible, daily. Walking is the necessary oil for the human machine.

Important acupuncture point: St 36.

Herbs: sideritis cretica, thymus vulgaris, rosmarinus officinalis, foeniculum vulgare, cistus creticus, hypericum perforatum, salvia officinalis, ocimum basilicum, origanum vulgare, urtica dioica, tilia europea, melissa officinalis, helichrysum stoehas, petroselinum sativum.

Example of herb prescription: infusion of cistus creticus.

Grandma's remedies: walk in nature where are aromatic herbs, e.g. rosmarinus officinalis, origanum vulgare, salvia officinalis, foeniculum vulgare, flowering lemon tree, flower orange tree. Alternatively have these aromatic herbs in your house and smell them several times a day. Smell rosmarinus officinalis, it may boost memory and help prevent Alzheimer's disease.

Toothache

It was a summer afternoon in 1993 when an aircraftman (soldier of the Air Force) visited me at the medical office of the military unit feeling acute pain due to a bad tooth. At that time I was the head doctor at the military unit of Vonitsa and the dentist had the day off. I had the patient sit in the dentist's chair and "examined" his teeth. The lightest pressure on his teeth brought terrible pain to the aircraftman.

I told him that there were three options; the first was to visit the nearest health center or hospital after calling to find out where there was a dentist; the second was to give you painkillers and anti-inflammatory drugs to relieve you until the dentist comes back; the third was to treat you with acupuncture and no matter you were relieved or not, the next morning you would visit the dentist.

He decided to have acupuncture and he asked if the needles hurt.

I inserted needles into the skin over the affected tooth (local painful points), dispersion and into LI 4, the sharp end of the needle was pointing towards the elbow, image 10, stimulation. He was immediately relieved and visited the dentist after a few days.

In case of toothache due to the back teeth at the upper jaw apart from the local painful points, I insert a needle at the point SI 1, stimulation.

In case of toothache due to the rest upper jaw teeth I insert needles at the local painful points and at point St 45.

In case of toothache due to the lower jaw teeth I insert needles at the local painful points and at LI 4, the sharp end of the needle should be pointing towards the elbow, stimulation.

Two years ago I visited the dentist because I was feeling awful when cold water touched the wisdom tooth at the lower right jaw or when I chewed food with the right back teeth. He told me that my wisdom tooth had chronic pulpitis and that I needed aponeurosis. "Is the aponeurosis urgent? I would prefer first to try acupuncture", I said. "It can be done anytime" he replied with an arrogant tone, too sure that I would visit him very soon. Fortunately I was proved to be right and it's been two years I have no discomfort.

I inserted acupuncture needles at the painful local skin points of the cheek, dispersion and at LI 4, stimulation. At the next session I used the local painful points, dispersion and the LI 1, stimulation. Next sessions I used the general cycle for the stimulation of the immune system along with the local painful points.

Important acupuncture points: LI 4, local painful skin points.

Herbs: thymus vulgaris, rosmarinus officinalis, cistus creticus, hypericum perforatum, origanum vulgare, allium sativum.

Example of herb prescription: infusion of cistus creticus.

Grandma's remedies:

a. fill your mouth with a mixture of boiled vinegar with salt and honey or with a mixture of vinegar and salt or with infusion of matricaria chamomilla or with infusion of hypericum perforatum.

b. put in the cavity of the tooth or on and around the tooth, cotton impregnated with melted garlic or milk from stem of ficus carica or with infusion of origanum vulgare or thymus vulgaris or rosemary, or salvia officinalis or hypericum perforatum or cistus creticus or with olive oil with oregano or common thyme or hypericym perforatum or rosemary or salvia officinalis or cistus creticus.

c. place on and around the bad tooth a mixture of three well crushed garlic cloves and a pinch of salt.

d. if you can't have access to a dentist for a long time, put in the tooth cavity a mixture of white marble glue with 2 drops of white cement and colored powder (optional) or put in pinus halepensis resin or a mixture of pinus halepensis resin with 3 drops of blue vitriol.

e. for gingivitis: fill your mouth with infusion of salvia officinalis or hypericum perforatum.

f. for periodontitis: fill your mouth with air or water or hypericum perforatum oil or infusion of salvia officinalis, 150 times, 3 times daily.

g. for periodontitis: put in a cup equal amounts of salt, honey and baking soda, add a little bit Ceylon cinnamon and rakee; mix it well and use this mixture to brush your teeth. Then fill your mouth with matricaria chamomilla with baking soda, p. 191, 20 times.

h. homemade toothpaste: put it in a cup equal amounts of salt, honey and baking soda and mix them well.

i. homemade mouthwash: matricaria chamomilla with baking soda, p. 291; g, h and i are from http://giatrosofia -bartzokas. blogspot.gr/.

j. homemade toothpaste: water with salt, in grams ratio 5: 1.

k. chew small olive tree leaves.

l. two days fasting.

Myopia, cataract

Myopia and cataract are not simple diseases. Try to treat them in the first stage.

I repeatedly use the point Gb 31, the sharp end of the needle should be pointing towards the knee, stimulation. Have patience.

Avoid TV, computer, night driving and places with intense light or polluted atmosphere.

Have sufficient light while reading; light direction should be from left for right handed and from right for the left handed.

Important acupuncture points: Gb 31, SJ 23.

Herbs: ruta graveolens, blueberry-vaccinium vitis idaea, thymus vulgaris, rosmarinus officinalis, helianthus annuus, matricaria chamomilla, chelidonium majus, anethum graveolens, urtica dioica, plantago major, veronica officinalis, lactuca sativa, carrot.

Examples of herb prescription:

a. infusion of 1/2 teaspoon ruta graveolens, 1-3 times daily.

b. infusion of rosmarinus officinalis.

c. drink 4 carrots juice, 2 times daily.

d. eat one handful raw sunflower seeds or sprouts.

Grandma's remedies for myopia:

a. keep your eyes moving fluidly for approximately 2 minutes for every hour you are on a screen or a computer.

b. exercise your eyes, it is very helpful: 1. focus on your thumb, firstly having your hand outstretched and then slowly bringing it to your nose, and then do the opposite hand movement. Repeat it 10 times. 2. look up towards your eyebrow and roll your eyes around in a circular motion as far as they can, in each direction. 3. look far away at an object for 10-15 seconds, then gaze at something close for 10-15 seconds. Then look back at the distant object. Repeat it 10 times.

c. blink often to moisten your eyes.

d. relax your eyes by placing your palms on the eyelids without pressing the eyes, for a few seconds.

e. put 3 drops lukewarm infusion of hyssopus officinalis in each eye.

f. boil 500g rosmarinus officinalis in 2 liters of water and pour it in the bathtub; enjoy your bath for 15 minutes.

g. walk outdoors and look far away.

Grandma's remedies for cataract:

a. put 1-2 drops of organic honey in the affected eye, 2 times daily.

b. put lukewarm pumpkin flower juice on the eyelids, 2 times daily.

c. eat a handful of bilberry or blueberry, daily.

d. put 3 drops of melilotus officinalis juice in the affected eye, once daily.

e. bake shells of stork egg, pound them well and from this powder add a little in the affected eye (monk Gymnasios Lavriotis).

f. apply a lukewarm mixture of equal parts of chelidonium majus juice (if you break the stems or leaves, you get thick juice) and honey on the eyelids; you might need to warm up the mixture. Apply it once daily.

g. eat 2-3 cloves of garlic daily.

h. eat spinach.

i. exercise your eyes, as mentioned above.

Burn, bedsore

Acupuncture will relieve your burning sensation immediately and will significantly minimize scarring because the local excess of energy, "fire", will be dispersed, "put out", in very short time. The key point is that the excess of energy will be dispersed not only from the surface but also from the deep skin layers.

I use local points peripherally to the burn, always at the healthy-unburned skin, dispersion and I insert needles at the corresponding finger/toe points (images 11, 12, 17, 18, 19, 20), stimulation. I immediately disperse the energy excess and activate-stimulate the "mechanisms for rehabilitation".

The needles that are inserted peripherally to the burn do not prevent you from applying any ointment (e.g. calendula) or herb oil on the burn.

In extensive or deep burns, seek for hospital immediately. While you are waiting for medical treatment, raise the injury above your heart. Don't get undressed, but make sure no clothing is stuck to the burn.

In bedsores I use acupuncture in exactly the same way.

Important acupuncture points: local peripheral points and the corresponding finger/toe points.

Herbs: plantago major, calendula officinalis, hypericum perforatum, matricaria chamomilla, helichrysum stoehas, aloe vera.

Example of herb prescription: infusion of plantago major.

Grandma's remedies for burns:

a. first degree burn (red, not blistered skin): apply on the burn cotton soaked with white spirit (or alcohol) or whipped raw egg whites (meringue) or a slice of raw potato or a slice of carrot. You can soak the wound in cool water for five minutes or longer.

b. second degree burn (extremely red, blistered skin and sore): apply linen cloth or bandage or cotton well soaked (it must be constantly wet) with white spirit (or alcohol) for half an hour; remove it and apply whipped raw egg whites (meringue) mixed with olive oil with hypericum perforatum or mixed with plain olive oil.
  In first and second degree burns you can apply ointments (or olive oils with the same herbs) of hypericum perforatum, calendula officinalis, arnica montana or a mixture of them or aloe vera gel.

Grandma's remedies for bedsores: apply olive oil with hypericum perforatum or ointment of hypericum perforatum.

If you want to use a product dermatologically tested, suitable for face, body and kids, compatible with homeopathy, without artificial colors, fragrance, parabens, PEGs, lanolin, silicones or mineral oils, I recommend **Think GAEA Calendula-Hypericum cream**.

It is used for:

• minor burns (solar and thermal), bedsores, ulcers and abrasions.

• conditions such as eczema, atopic dermatitis, psoriasis.

The beneficial properties of Think GAEA are based on the supercritical herbal extracts, extra virgin olive oil (antioxidant) and beeswax (softening and moisturizing effect).

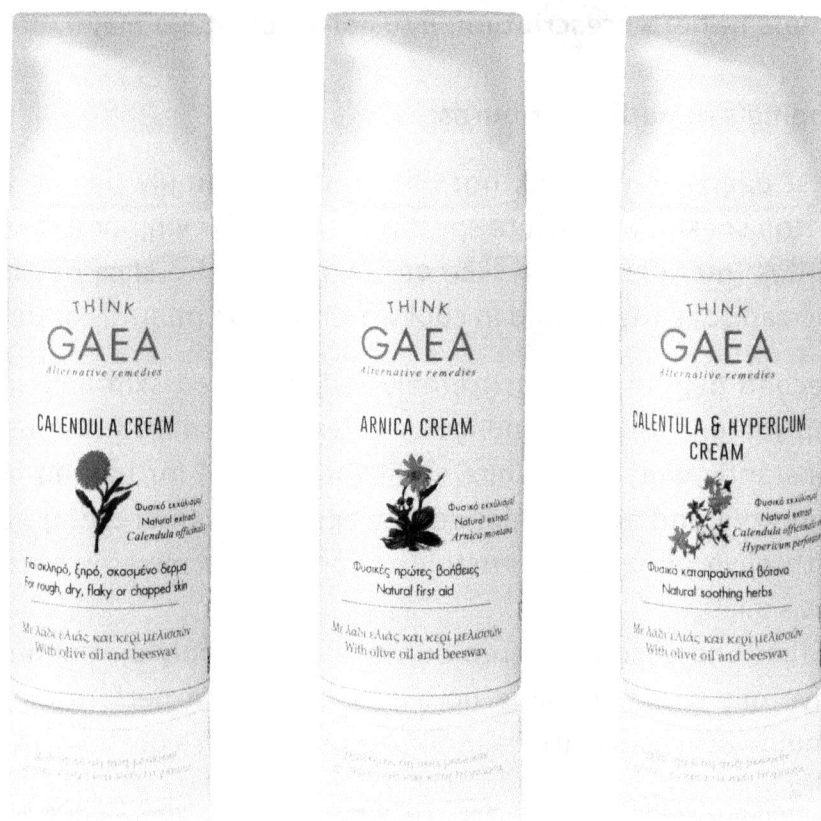

Think GAEA Calendula cream is ideal for tired, dry, rough, chapped skin.

Calendula officinalis, traditionally used for its multiple soften-ing properties, provides intense hydration and soothes irritation.

It is used:
- for light sunburns, redness and mild irritation.
- for hand treatment, care and hydration of damaged skin.
- in eczema, atopic dermatitis, rash.
- as a nappy rash cream.

Think GAEA
45 Artemidos, 16343
Ilioupolis, Athens
Greece
www.think gaea.com   info@thinkgaea.gr

Varicose veins

Tired and swollen legs with enlarged veins can be relieved with acupuncture. I use a needle at St 36, the sharp end of the needle should be pointing towards the abdomen, dispersion. You will feel your legs relaxed from the first session and you will continue to acupuncture. If you apply acupuncture more than twice a week, insert the needle perpendicular to the skin.

Point St 36, dispersion, is the best choice for all those people whose feet hurt after long hours of standing.

Do the homemade spa by adding coarse salt in the bathtub or put your feet in a basin filled with salty water; the water should be at a temperature of your choice.

Exercise regularly, walking in shallow waters, can help to re-duce the appearance and effects of varicose veins. A lot of people choose to wear supportive compression socks.

Important acupuncture point: St 36.

Herbs: rosmarinus officinalis, crategus oxyacantha, ruscus aculeatus, hypericum perforatum, verbascum thapsus, melilotus officinalis, aesculus hippocastanum, achillea millefolium, allium sativum, calendula officinalis, tilia europea.

Examples of herb prescription:

 a. infusion of ruscus aculeatus, 2 times daily.

b. infusion of melilotus officinalis.

Grandma's remedies:

a. apply an ointment of a mixture of hypericum perforatum, verbascum thapsus and ruta graveolens.

b. boil 50g oak bark in 1 L water for 15 minutes. Add it in the bathtub; you can also massage your legs using this decoction.

Constipation

Constipation is a common problem of people living in the developed countries. Stress, a low fiber diet, not drinking enough fluids, ignoring the urge to go to defecate, a lack of exercise, certain medications and supplements, hormonal disorders and medical conditions are the main causes of constipation.

To help you realize the magnitude of the problem of constipation I will give you the example of a factory that can not reject its waste. The immediate result is dysfunction and the final is factory closure. In humans, the failure of rejection of faeces creates internal intoxication which, according to hygienists, is the cause of many diseases.

Some gastroenterologists consider it normal to defecate a few hours after each meal. Others consider 3 to 21 bowel movements a week as normal. Many gastroenterologists consider that constipation is the need to strain to have a bowel movement or the experience of a feeling of incomplete elimination after a bowel movement.

Acupuncture can effectively help both for anxiety, p. 119 and for mobilization of the intestine. I use points St 36, the sharp end of the needle should be pointing towards the toes, stimulation and St 25, which is located 8-10cm bilateral to the navel, image 8. The needle is inserted perpendicular to the skin, stimulation.

You should establish a time each day to use the bathroom. Stay in the bathroom for up to 15 minutes, don't strain to have a bowel movement.

Proper diet with plenty of fiber (vegetables, fruit, nuts, pulses, unrefined cereals, sprouts, olive oil and olives), relaxation and exercise are necessary.

Important acupuncture points: St 36, St 25.

Herbs: linseed, origanum majorana, stigmata maydis (zea mays hairs), thymus vulgaris, foeniculum vulgare, ocimum basilicum, salvia officinalis, origanum vulgare, taraxacum officinalis, cichorium intibus, wild rose, hypericum perforatum, melissa officinalis, pimpinella anisum, rubus fruticosus, mentha piperata, mentha spicata, achillea millefolium, artemisia vulgaris, angelica archangelica, cassia angustifolia, almond tree, plantago major, prune, fig, hot pepper

Examples of herb prescription:

a. add 1 tablespoon of pounded linseeds in your food or water, 2 times daily.

b. infusion of origanum majorana.

c. drink 100ml of stigmata maydis (zea mays hairs) infusion, 2 times daily.

Grandma's remedies:

a. drink a cup of warm water mixed with 1 teaspoon of honey, every morning.

b. drink the water of a glass where 3 prunes or figs were soaked for 10 hours and eat the prunes or figs.

c. eat a handful of almonds or walnuts or peanuts and 1 dried fig, daily.

d. eat wholegrain bread instead of white.

e. eat meals which have fibers and try the fibers to be equally shared.

f. reduce sugar intake, replace it with fresh or dried fruit (banana, lotus, melon, watermelon, mango, kiwi, cherries, strawberry, pear, grapes, apple, ripe orange or tangerine).

Hemorrhoids

Hemorrhoids are a direct result of constipation and a consequence of the same causes.

I use the points for constipation along with Gb 41 which is located 4cm from the gap between the small and the fourth toe, images 13, 22. The sharp end of the needle should be pointing towards the ankle, dispersion.

Change your diet, avoid alcohol, spicy and savory dishes, drink enough fluids, apply the raw food diet, treat constipation, deal with your stress, exercise and have sitz baths, p. 83.

Important acupuncture point: Gb 41

Herbs: hypericum perforatum, verbascum undulatum, arum maculatum, urtica dioica, achillea millefolium, calendula officinalis, plantago major, ranunculus ficaria, ruscus aculeatus, ganoderma lucidum, rosmarinus officinalis.

Examples of herb prescription:

a. infusion of hypericum perforatum.

b. arum maculatum, p. 70.

c. infusion of ranunculus ficaria.

Grandma's remedies:

a. apply ointment of a mixture of hypericum perforatum, verbascum undulatum and ruta graveolens.

b. apply ointment of a mixture of hypericum perforatum, achillea millefolium, plantago major and calendula officinalis.

c. apply pulp of rosmarinus officinalis flowering tops (use blender).

d. apply powder of dried stalks of eggplant.

e. apply pulp of petroselinum sativum (use blender).

f. wash locally with infusion of 3 teaspoons urtica dioica.

g. wash locally with oak bark or ulmus minor bark decoction.

h. cut a finger from a plastic glove, poor water into and close it with a thread; place it in the freezer. When it's frozen, use it for the internal hemorrhoids.

i. exercise: suck inwards your belly and stay for a while in this position, relax and repeat.

j. fruit-therapy for 7 days (e.g. eat only watermelon).

Hair Loss

Usually acupuncture is effective to stop losing your hair. If you are distressed, relaxed and you have physical improvement, then you will reverse hair loss.

I use the points for relaxation, p. 119 and I apply the general cycle for the stimulation of the immune system, p. 123.

Relax, try self-hypnosis. It is important to stop eating sweet foods.

Important acupuncture points: St 36, SP 1, SP 4, CV 17.

Herbs: adiantum capillus-veneris, rosmarinus officinalis, laurus nobillis, salvia officinalis, psoralea bituminosa, juglans regia, asplenium ceterach, hypericum perforatum, matricaria chamomilla, tilia europea, melissa officinalis, allium sativum, urtica dioica, thymus vulgaris.

Examples of herb prescription: infusion of adiantum capillus-veneris or rosmarinus officinalis or laurus nobillis.

Grandma's remedies:

a. first shampoo your hair and rinse; then for 5 minutes massage using infusion of adiantum capillus-veneris or rosmarinus officinalis or laurus nobillis or salvia officinalis and don't rinse. This remedy also helps in dandruff.

b. first shampoo your hair and rinse; then apply to your head a mixture of honey and water in a volume ratio of 1: 4, leave it for 15 minutes and rinse using plenty of water.

c. first shampoo your hair and rinse; then massage using olive oil or olive oil with laurus nobillis or olive oil with hypericum per-foratum; leave it for 15 minutes; shampoo your hair and rinse again. Repeat it every other day.

d. drink 60ml beetroot juice, 3 times daily.

e. for local alopecia:

1. rub the area with a peeled and cut garlic clove.
2. rub the area with milk from silybum marianum stem until skin becomes pink, once daily.
3. put an ivory button in little lemon juice for 12 hours, so as to melt; then apply it, once a day.

Calus, wart

The calluses on the soles go away easily if you insert needles right at their center for 10 days, once daily. Usually the points at the center of the calluses hurt, but the result will reward you. When the calluses disappear, you will feel better not only at your feet, but throughout your body because the calluses are caused by en-ergy imbalance which is corrected by the needles.

Avoid closed and tight shoes.

For warts I use any point just peripheral to the wart at the unaf-fected skin. If you have multiple, apply the general cycle for the stimulation of the immune system, p. 123, along with one of the relaxation points, p. 119.

Important acupuncture points: a point at the center of callus and any point peripheral to the wart.

Herbs: sideritis cretica, allium sativum, melissa officinalis, olea europea, hypericum perforatum, salvia officinalis, matricaria chamomilla, tilia europea.

Example of herb prescription: infusion of sideritis cretica.

Grandma's remedies:

a. put a peeled garlic clove in aluminum foil in the oven and bake it. Warm-soft, apply it (without aluminum foil) on the callus and stabilize it with a bandage overnight. Probably the same morning or the next (repeat it) the callus will disappear or become detached and you can pull it out using tweezers.

b. place on callus a slice of lemon or tomato or pineapple bark and stabilize it with a bandage overnight. Probably the same morning or the next (repeat it) the callus will disappear or become detached and you can pull it out using tweezers.

c. for wart and callus: apply milk drops from ficus carica stalk or calendula officinalis stem, 4 times daily.

d. apply on warts pinus halepensis resin, 2 times daily.

Dysmenorrhea (painful periods)

Help yourself using the point SP 4, the sharp end of the needle should be pointing towards the ankle, stimulation. In next sessions apply the general cycle for the stimulation of the immune system, p. 123 and use one of relaxation points, p. 119.

As always, you should visit a medical doctor at least once. Women should wear clothes that cover-warm the entire abdomen.

Important acupuncture point: SP 4.

Herbs: melissa officinalis, salvia officinalis, origanum vulgare, matricaria chamomilla, tilia europea, viburnum opulus, valeriana officinalis, achillea millefolium, urtica dioica, trigonella foenum graecum, rosmarinus officinalis, petroselinum sativum, lycopus europaeus, ruta graveolens.

Example of herb prescription: infusion of melissa officinalis.

Grandma's remedies: apply on the abdomen olive oil with common sage or chamomile.

Eczema (atopic dermatitis), psoriasis

Eczema is usually an itchy skin condition of unknown aetiology apart from eczema due to contact with dye, varnish and other chemicals. It is characterized by itchy, erythematous, vesicular, weeping and crusting patches. The skin hardens, loses its elasticity, its color changes (becomes a mix of white, brown, pink) and there are cracks (which go beyond the stratum corneum) which may bleed slightly.

If you apply cortisone ointment on the eczema, there is immediate improvement; the cracks close and the skin surface becomes smooth. The effect of steroid ointments is temporary and the eczema returns in worse condition. You are forced to use stronger steroid creams (one always should start with first generation

steroid cream and finally ends up with the strong latest generation) and become trapped in a chronic vicious cycle.

If you use these ointments, you should really put a minimum
amount (there's no need to create a layer of ointment on the eczema); most importantly try not to ever start the cortisone or try
to get away from it. You should start by applying some fat cream,
or olive oil (from the vigil candle of a Saint preferably), or chamomile compress, 4 times daily; also apply healthy diet (light meals)
and thermal baths. The steroid ointments should be a last resort
for you.

Acupuncture will help you. In both eczema and psoriasis I apply
the allergy prevention, p. 181.

When you feel itchy and want to scrape yourself, don't do it;
insert a needle at St 36, the sharp end of the needle should be
pointing towards the abdomen, dispersion, image 22. It is important not to scrape yourself because the skin gets worse.

In contact eczema insert needles as I described in allergy countryside, p. 180.

Drink plenty of fluids, avoid foods that are sweet, salty and
spicy, apply the relaxation methods, p. 12, have thermal baths and
do not come into contact with irritants (detergents etc.). If your
dermatologist is not sure that the dermatitis is eczema, then get
a biopsy.

The most important treatment in eczema and psoriasis is the
inner detoxification of thoughts.

Important acupuncture points: St 36, SP 4.

Herbs: cistus creticus, urtica dioica, thymus vulgaris, calendula officinalis, silybum marianum, plantago major, avena sativa, taraxacum officinalis, matricaria chamomilla, melissa officinalis, hypericum perforatum, aloe vera, juglans regia, origanum vulgare, viola

tricolor, rosmarinus officinalis, salvia officinalis, gallium aparine, arctium lappa, symphytum officinale.

Example of herb prescription: infusion of cistus creticus.

Grandma's remedies:

a. apply ointment of one of the above mentioned herbs or a mixture of some of them.

b. if you feel itchy apply chamomile with baking soda, p. 191.

c. in psoriasis: apply a cotton soaked with chamomile with baking soda, p. 191, for 10 minutes. Then massage using a mixture of 1 tablespoon honey and 1 tablespoon baking soda (well mixed until they become cream) for 10 minutes. Wash the affected skin using boiled chamomile with baking soda, p. 191 and massage again with the above mentioned mixture. Repeat the same process for 1 hour. Then apply an ointment made from olive oil and bee wax, p. 53. Do it until psoriasis disappears, once daily. The b and c are from http://giatrosofia -bartzokas.blogspot.gr/.

Acne

"Doctor, I can not stand my pimples anymore; I feel that everyone is looking at my pimples; I feel that no boy likes me."

If the pimples are all over the face, I insert a needle at St 36, the sharp end of the needle should be pointing towards the abdomen, dispersion, image 22.

If the pimples are only on the forehead, I insert a needle at LU 5, the sharp end of the needle should be pointing towards the shoulder, dispersion, image 9.

If the pimples are found only on the chin, I insert a needle at Liv 3, which is located 1cm above the union of great and second toe, image 13. The sharp end of the needle should be pointing towards the ankle, stimulation.

If the pimples are on the cheeks, I insert a needle at St 36, the sharp end of the needle should be pointing towards the abdomen, dispersion.

Apart from these points, I use each relaxation acupoint, p. 119, alternately.

In next sessions I apply the general cycle for the stimulation of the immune system, at point St 36 I insert the needle perpendicularly.

In case of remaining scars I use the general cycle for the stimulation of the immune system along with LU 5 and a relaxation acupoint.

Try not to squeeze your pimples, especially with dirty hands. After squeezing a pimple, rub gently using a fresh lemon slice for sterilization at least 6 times a day for 3 days.

Avoid sweets and anything sweetened, remember fruit therapy and raw food diet. Wash your face with soap (with neutral pH) and water, at least 3 times a day. Use the relaxation methods, p. 12.

Important acupuncture points: St 36, LU 5, Liv 3.

Herbs: calendula officinalis, thymus vulgaris, allium sativum, cistus creticus, sideritis cretica, petroselinum sativum, urtica dioica, silybum marianum, plantago major, taraxacum officinalis, matricaria chamomilla, melissa officinalis, aloe vera, tomato, juglans regia, origanum vulgare, rosmarinus officinalis, salvia officinalis, symphytum officinale.

Example of herb prescription: infusion of calendula officinalis.

Grandma's remedies:

a. wash your face well using decoction of petroselinum sativum, 3 times daily.

b. apply, on washed face, a slice of organic tomato for 15 minutes, wash out thoroughly, 2 times daily.

c. apply on your face water in which burnt iron has been extinguished (monk Gymnasios Lavriotis).

d. wash the skin with boiled chamomile and baking soda, p. 191. Mix well equal quantities of honey, baking soda and Ceylon cinnamon until it becomes creamy and apply it on acne. The longer stays, the better. Wash out with boiled chamomile and baking soda, p. 191, http://giatrosofia -bartzokas.blogspot.gr/.

Insomnia

Insomnia is a sleeping disorder characterized by the inability to sleep and/or the inability to remain asleep as long as desired and often it is described as an experience of non-refreshing sleep.

Acupuncture is an effective therapy for insomnia. When I can't sleep I use the point Extra 1, dispersion. The result is usually immediate and of course I don't wake up to remove the needle.

If you suffer from insomnia, insert a needle at each acupoint for relaxation, p. 119, alternately, once daily. Remember point SJ 5 for depression. I sometimes also use St 36, dispersion, so as to move the energy from the head (where it is in excess) towards the legs. The same action has point Gb 41, the sharp end of the needle should be pointing towards the ankle, dispersion, image 13.

The most beneficial sleep hours are between 23.00 to 03.00. The prerequisite for an easy and rejuvenating sleep is to free our mind from conscious and subconscious thoughts. Apply one of the methods of relaxation, p. 12, daily. if you have toxic persistent worries about earning money, personal ambitions or other selfish purposes, then you also have sleep problem. Our body can't rest without the pause of our thoughts.

If you can't escape from persistent annoying thoughts then visit a psychiatrist or find a dedicated priest and have confession-repentance.

Do not watch TV two hours before bedtime, just read a pleasant book.

Do not eat 3 hours before going to bed.

Do not drink coffee or stimulant beverages (e.g. type cola).

Treat constipation.

Do not sleep in the afternoon and do not wake up late in the morning.

Exercise every day, walk in nature.

Avoid intense fatigue before bedtime, mild respiratory exercises are recommended.

Have sexual intercourse with your beloved person (energy exchange), it is an excellent sleeping pill.

Remove the phone from your head, turn off (not just disable) the electronic devices in your room.

If you have bright colored (e.g. red, yellow, orange) bedroom walls, change them using a gentle pal color.

The room temperature should be around 20°C and well ventilated. Have light and warm blankets in winter.

Wear comfortable, not tight, pajamas.

Your bedroom should have continuous ventilation which provides fresh air in your lungs and good oxygenation of your brain.

There are patients suffering from sleep apnea syndrome, usually obese; when they get awake, they feel tired and exhausted. A visit to a pulmonologist is required. They should lose weight and possibly place a special mask during sleep. Acupuncture helps, use points St 9, bilaterally, dispersion, LI 20, unilaterally, dispersion, LU 5, dispersion and CV 17, dispersion.

If underground earth rays intersect at a terrestrial point, usually because of running underground water, then this point is morbid to humans. If your bed (or seat in your workplace) is located at this point, you will be affected by geopathical radiation all night long for years, with the result of insomnia, headache, leukemia, Parkinson's disease, multiple sclerosis, stomach bleeding, arteriosclerosis, arthritis, epilepsy, depression, cancer, etc. . Geopathical radiation may also explain the case of houses which have the reputation of being cursed and their interchangeable residents die.

Before buying a house and placing the bed or the desk, check for geopathical radiation.

One way to check the position of your bed, desk or the location to build your house is to apply the muscle test for selecting food-substances, p. 30.

Apply the test at the place of bed, desk, or location of your future house. If your hands withstand the soft power of an examiner, then the places are safe. If at the point you already have your bed, your hands fall, then move it in another place. There are experts who place appropriate minerals to neutralize the geopathical radiation.

Do not build houses near high-voltage lines.

Important acupuncture point: Extra 1.

Herbs: matricaria chamomilla, melissa officinalis, tilia europea, valeriana officinalis, passiflora incarnata, hypericum perforatum, origanum vulgare, origanum majorana, rosmarinus officinalis, salvia officinalis, mentha spicata, ocimum basilicum, lactuca sativa, olea europea, petroselinum sativum, lavandula officinalis.

Example of herb prescription: infusion of matricaria chamomilla, 4 times daily.

Grandma's remedies:

a. infusion of a mixture of melissa officinalis and origanum majorana.

b. infusion of a mixture of salvia officinalis, mentha spicata, petroselinum sativum and agropyron repens.

c. boil a whole lettuce in 1/2 L water for 10 minutes. Drink 1 teacup before bedtime.

d. change the atmosphere of your bedroom by placing herbs as common thyme, savory, rosemary, common sage, basil, oregano.

e. drink a glass of warm milk with honey before bedtime.

Snoring

Before having surgery, acupuncture yourself.

I use the points:

St 9, bilaterally, the sharp end of the needle should be pointing towards the head, dispersion.

LU 5, the sharp end of the needle should be pointing towards the shoulder, dispersion.

LI 4, the sharp end of the needle should be pointing towards the elbow, stimulation.

Possibly snoring will recede immediately; for permanent results you will need several sessions. Sleep on your right side.

Lose weight if you are overweight.

Avoid heavy dinners, stop smoking and abstain from alcohol. Have your nose decongested.

Important acupuncture points: St 9, LU 5.

Herbs: satureja thymbra, thymus vulgaris, salvia officinalis, sideritis cretica, althea officinalis, plantago major, hypericum perforatum, tilia europea, melissa officinalis.

Example of herb prescription: infusion of sideritis cretica.

Grandma's remedy: infusion of salvia officinalis before bedtime.

Prostatic hypertrophy

Before you have an operation or even better when the first symptoms of prostatic hypertrophy appear (decrease of the radius of urination, difficulty at initiating urination and the need for urinating during the night), start acupuncture and herbal therapy.

I use Bl 57, the sharp end of the needle should be pointing towards the abdomen, dispersion and the local point which is located one centimeter above the root of the penis, image 8, dispersion. The sharp end of the needle should be pointing towards the abdomen and should **never** puncture the skin of the penis. The results will surprise you pleasantly.

You may also have sitz baths therapy, p. 83.

Important acupuncture points: Bl 57, local point.

Herbs: hypericum perforatum, urtica dioica, cistus creticus, arctostaphylos uva ursi, agropyron repens, stigmata maydis (zea mays hairs), platanus fructus tot, serenoa repens (saw palmetto, sabal serrulatan), glycyrrhiza glabra, petroselinum sativum, pumkin, watermelon, almond tree, arbutus officinalis, equisetum arvense, melissa officinalis, asplenium ceterach, plantago major, epilodium parviflorum, apium graveolens, pinus halepensis, eryngium campestre, origanum majorana, lippia citriodora, rosmarinus officinalis, pistacia lentiscus var. chia, lemon, cynara cardunculus, salvia officinalis.

Examples of herb prescription: infusion of hypericum perforatum or urtica dioica or cistus creticus.

Grandma's remedies:

a. boil 6 platanus fructus tot in 1 L water for 15 minutes. Drink 1 glass of it every morning.

b. decoction of a mixture of 33% urtica dioica roots, 33% serenoa repens (saw palmetto-sabal serrulatan), 17% stigmata maydis (zea mays hairs) and 17% arctostaphylos uva ursi.

c. infusion of a mixture of asplenium ceterach and plantago major, 2 times daily.

d. boil 7 artichokes in 1 L of water. Drink 1 glass from the mixture of artichokes juice with decoction of agropyron repens roots and a teaspoon olive oil, 2 times daily.

e. if you suffer from calf pain, apply olive oil with chamomilla or hypericum perforatum or cistus creticus on the calf. Sometimes calf pain indicates prostate disorder.

f. apply hypericum perforatum or urtica dioica or cistus creticus ointment on the penis root and the perineum (the area between the anus and testicles), 4 times daily.

Breast tumors

The most recent data indicate that women who reach the age of 35 should undergo a mammography. Gynecologists point out that women after the age of 40 should undergo every year an imaging evaluation of the breasts.

Preventive gynecological check is invaluable. If you have any formation in the chest and you treat it conservatively with regular monitoring by tests (ultrasound, mammography, CT, MRI) or if you have a rather benign formation and want to avoid surgery (if the doctor gives you a two-month period before the biopsy or surgery), then the extra treatment that you can offer yourself is acupuncture.

You can do the same if you have had a surgery for breast cancer.

Two are the important points:

St 18 which is located in the groove under the breast on the imaginary vertical line passing through the nipple of the breast, image 8. The sharp end of the needle should be pointing towards the head, dispersion.

Pc 6, stimulation, the sharp end of the needle should be pointing towards the fingers.

If you have a malignant tumor, then after the surgical removal you can do acupuncture (before surgery you can also do acupuncture to stimulate the immune system, help the respiratory system and to relax). Find an acupuncturist that will show you at which points you can insert needles and certainly remember the points for relaxation, p. 119.

Important acupuncture points: St 18, Pc 6.

Herbs, Examples of herb prescription and Grandma's remedies:

same as those of cancer, p. 151. In case of benign cysts the same as those of relaxation, p. 119. You should also try (do the muscle test for selecting food-substances): thymus vulgaris, gallium aparine, lonicera japonica.

Spinal cord injury
(paraparesis, paraplegia, tetraparesis, quadriplegia)

In the U.S. each year there are 10,000 new cases of spinal cord injuries, with a total of 200,000 patients and a $ 4 billion per year cost (survey of 1992).

Spinal cord injury means that there is reduced or no mobility or sensation in limbs with impaired urination and defecation.

If a similar accident happens in your wider environment, apart from the organized hospital, it would be advisable to visit a qualified acupuncturist.

There is an article in the Journal of Traditional Chinese Medicine 16 (2): 134-137, 1996, with the title "Acupuncture Treatment of Complete Traumatic Paraplegia". It is an analysis of 261 cases (261 patients with complete paraplegia after injury, treated with acupuncture); 8 patients (3.1%) were actually treated, 92 patients (35.2%) were significantly improved, 149 (57.1%) patients were improved and 12 patients (5%) had no improvement. The overall efficiency was 95%. The authors in their final comments suggest that acupuncture should be applied as soon as possible so that the regenerative process of the nervous tissue is more likely to be successful.

There are articles claiming that acupuncture improves spinal cord swelling: Unfallchirurgie 1983 Dec; 9 (6): 308-13, J. Altern Complement Med. 2002 Jun; 8 (3): 341-9. When the swelling of the first days improves, then more nerve cells survive resulting in less disability.

As an initial and immediate therapy, three needles should be inserted: the first in the back, in the midline, on the spot-level of the damage (spinal cord injury), the second needle at acupuncture point N 1 and the third at CV 17 for relaxation.

Caution: you must not move the spine (neck, back, lumbar) of a patient with spinal cord injury or possible spinal cord injury after an accident.

In paraplegics I do the same acupuncture as in cerebral stroke but I insert needles only in lower extremities, alternately. Needles at all points should be inserted perpendicular to the skin.

Important acupuncture points: local point in the midline of the spine on the spot of the damage, Kd 1, CV 17.

Herbs: hypericum perforatum, rosmarinus officinalis, avena sativa, verbena officinalis, satureja thymbra, thymus vulgaris.

Example of herb prescription: infusion of hypericum perforatum.

Grandma's remedy: do self-hypnosis, replacing the injured spinal cord with the healthy spinal cord that you had at an earlier age, e.g. when you were five years old.

Multiple sclerosis (demyelinating disease)

It is the second most common cause of neurological disability among young people; the first is spinal cord injury.

It is an inflammation and destruction of myelin (sheath of axons) of the central nervous system (brain and spinal cord). The cause of the disease, as in most degenerative chronic diseases, is unknown. There is, however, an impaired immune system.

Apply 3 times the general cycle for the stimulation of the immune system, p. 123 along with acupuncture for relaxation, p. 119. Then apply the general cycle for the stimulation of the kidneys, p. 160.

Remember the general advice for prayer, cleansing the soul (confession, repentance), consuming pure food, fasting, fruit therapy, exercise and thermal baths.

It is worth fighting, do not surrender to the disease, but fight with faith, patience and love towards the Creator.

Important acupuncture points: St 36, CV 17.

Herbs: cistus creticus, hypericum perforatum, thymus vulgaris, satureja thymbra, salvia officinalis, rosmarinus officinalis, avena sativa, verbena officinalis, urtica dioica, oxalis pes caprae, matricaria chamomilla.

Example of herb prescription: infusion of cistus creticus.

Grandma's remedies:

a. hydrogen peroxide, p. 156.

b. massage the weak extremities using olive oil with chamomile.

Heart diseases, cholesterol

It's winter time, the cold is bitter and a man around fifties after a heavy dinner comes out of a restaurant in a very bad spirit and looks thoughtful and pale. With difficulty ascends the road and unfortunately collapses.

In case of heart diseases you visit a cardiologist, just as for other diseases you address to the proper medical doctor.

Acupuncture helps for heart diseases but you should address to a specialist.

In general I am addressing to patients in remote places without health assistance.

Two are the points you can use in case of heart pain waiting for medical help: CV 17 and Pc 6. You can also use Extra 1 for antistressing.

Little food, relaxation, walking, control of cholesterol, glucose, blood pressure and constipation, avoidance of bad habits (smoke, alcohol, caffeine, stimulating substances, overindulgence of sex) are preventive and therapeutic measures.

For cholesterol control apart from eating carefully, exercising and relaxation I recommend:

Important acupuncture points: St 36, CV 17.

Herbs: olea europea, allium sativum, portulaca oleracea, curcuma longa, crategus oxyacantha, cynara cardunculus, taraxacum officinale, trigonella foenum graecum, tilia europea, pistacia lentiscus var. chia, melissa officinalis, goji berry, rosmarinus officinalis, honey with cinnamomum zeylanicum, hot pepper, raphanus sativus, helichrysum stoehas.

Example of herb prescription: infusion of taraxacum officinale.

Grandma's remedies:

a. eat 4 unsalted olives, daily

b. cover the bottom of a glass with pistacia lentiscus var. chia crystals, fill the glass with water and the next morning drink only the water. Refill it with water and after 24 hours drink the water. Repeat this process for 2 months. In 30 days replace the pistacia lentiscus var. chia crystals.

c. decoction of a mixture of olea europea and rosmarinus officinalis, 2 times daily.

d. eat a mixture of 1 teaspoon honey and ½ teaspoon cinnamomum zeylanicum, 2 times daily.

e. after finishing a meal have 1 radish.

Precaution saves lives especially of young people. Instead of
stressing ourselves for what we have or want to keep or for more
possessions, we should thank God because we are healthy, can
breathe freely, walk and enjoy life.

Important acupuncture points: Pc 6, CV 17.

Herbs: crategus oxyacantha, tilia europea, allium sativum, leonurus cardiaca, viscum album, cistus creticus, satureja thymbra,
mentha spicata, achillea millefolium, hypericum perforatum, thymus vulgaris, salvia officinalis, rosmarinus officinalis, valeriana
officinalis, viburnum opulus, urtica dioica, olea europea, althea
officinalis, melissa officinalis.

Example of herb prescription: infusion of 2 teaspoons crategus
oxyacantha little leaves, blossoms or fruit, 3 times daily for a long
time.

Grandma's remedies:

a. if you are under heart attack firstly be calm, secondly ask for
help, thirdly take 2 aspirins which don't affect the stomach, in
case you don't have aspirins place under your tongue a piece of
garlic clove, fourthly breathe deeply 2-3 times and don't start
coughing.

b. in case of irregular heart beatings drink infusion of leonurus cardiaca 3 times daily. The authentic almond milk (soumada), p. 35 with water and little honey helps. Infusion of crategus oxyacantha or melissa officinalis or orange tree blossoms or valeriana officinalis or mentha spicata are helpful as well.

c. herbs with antithrombotic action: allium sativum, melilotus officinalis, aesculus hippocastanum.

d. hydrogen peroxide, p. 156.

e. fasting for 7 days or 14 days with fruit juice only.

Arthritis

As always you should visit a medical doctor; in this case a rheumatologist or GP. If the classical medicine fails or you do not want or can not get drugs, then take your fate into your own hands.

There are many types of arthritis, so there are many different ways of acupuncture.

I arbitrarily divide arthritis into monarticular and polyarthritis. When multiple joints hurt (polyarthritis), then I use 6 (3 points bilaterally means 6) points: SP 4, the sharp end of the needle should be pointing towards the big toe, dispersion, St 36, the sharp end of the needle should be pointing towards the abdomen, dispersion and SJ 5, the sharp end of the needle should be pointing towards the middle finger of the hand, dispersion. I insert a needle in any one of these 6 points alternately. During the same session I also use CV 17 or Pc 6 alternately. If the symptoms are not acute, I insert needles every other day for the first 2 weeks and then every three days.

When there is monoarticular arthritis, I use local painful points on the joint. If you feel pain deeply in the joint and you can not understand where the local painful points are, then I select painful points peripherally to the joint. I also exploit the corresponding points located half a centimeter below the nail angle of the fingers/toes depending on the inflamed area (images 11, 12, 17, 18, 19, 20). If the symptoms don't recede, I use the points mentioned in polyarthritis.

If polyarthritis and acute (severe pain, swelling, redness, stiffness) monoarticular arthritis coexist, insert needles for polyarthritis and monoarticular arthritis simultaneously.

Control your weight, drink enough water and follow the Mediterranean diet, p. 47.

Joint immobilization is beneficial in acute arthritis but progressive mobilization and exercising is helpful for chronic arthritis.

Remember the thermal baths and the recipe for homemade spa bath, p. 80.

Important acupuncture points: for polyarthritis SP 4, St 36, SJ 5, for monoarticular arthritis, local points and the corresponding finger/toe points.

Herbs: cistus creticus, hypericum perforatum, urtica dioica, allium sativum, arum maculatum, sideritis cretica, thymus vulgaris, origanum vulgare, olea europea, salix alba, allium cepa, potato, crategus oxyacantha, curcuma longa.

Examples of herb prescription: infusion of cistus creticus or urtica dioica.

Grandma's remedies:

a. around 1971 my aunt P. T. suffering from persistent rheumatic pains in the ribs and lower abdomen visited the physician Mr. Kokaraki in Athens, Skoufa street and was recommended to drink three aspirins 4 times a day, a total of 12 aspirins per day, for 7 days. The aspirins were dissolved in 100 ml water with half a teaspoon of baking soda and half a teaspoon of sugar. I should draw attention to the fact that my aunt had also stomach discomfort such as pain and heartburn and we know that aspirin is a cause of gastrointestinal bleeding.

She was also told to have bath with the hottest water she could tolerate. The results were impressive from the first day, the symptoms disappeared and until now she hasn't suffered from rheumatic pains again.

b. if you are relieved by hot pad, apply hot (tolerable) olive oil with oregano or common thyme or garlic or hypericum perforatum. If you are relieved by cold pad, apply olive oil with chamomile or tilia europea or urtica dioica or plain olive oil several times a day. You can cover the joint with transparent food film to avoid the clothes to get oiled. Instead of oil you can use the similar ointment. Two minutes prior to oil or ointment application you may massage gently the joint with white spirit or rakee.

c. crush well 3 whole peeled garlics and apply them on the joint, use a bandage to wrap the joint, leave it for 8 hours.

d. boil 1kg peeled crushed garlic in 1 L olive oil. Strain the olive oil and add 150g turpentine and 5 egg yolks; Mix them well and apply the mixture on the suffering joint.

e. in a cup put a teaspoon of hippophae seeds, a teaspoon of 1 crushed wild rose blossom, 5 hibiscus sabdariffa leaves and a little of crocus sativus. Pour really hot water in the cup, after 10 minutes drink it and eat the hippophae seeds, 2 times daily http://giatrosofia -bartzokas.blogspot.gr/.

f. hydrogen peroxide, p. 156.

g. if weather changes cause you joint pain, massage gently point

SJ 5 for 10 minutes or insert a needle, dispersion, the sharp end of the needle should be pointing towards the middle finger of the hand.

h. dissolve 1 teaspoon of Ceylon cinnamon powder and 2 teaspoons of honey in a glass of hot water, drink it, 2 times daily.

i. if you suffer from polyarthritis, 7 days of fasting or 14 days of fruit therapy will be helpful.

j. in gout, control serum uric acid by dietary restriction of meat, fatty cheese, seafood and alcohol. Drink enough water and check the diuretic intake.

Herbs for hyperuricemia: apium graveolens root, urtica dioica, acorus calamus, tilia europea, jasminum officinale, petroselinum sativum, potato, taraxacum officinalis, satureja thymbra, sambucus nigra, cherries stems, strawberries, teucrium chamaedrys, glycyrrhiza glabra.

Examples of herb prescription for hyperuricemia:

a. infusion of 2 teaspoons urtica dioica.

b. infusion of 2 teaspoons crategus oxyacantha small leaves, blossoms or fruit.

Grandma's remedies for hyperuricemia:

a. eat apium graveolens root every day.

b. drink a mixture of 240ml water, 1/2 teaspoon baking soda and 50ml lemon juice.

c. drink a mixture of 300ml water and 1/2 teaspoon baking soda. The maximum dose is 8 such mixtures per day. The baking soda increases blood pressure, so if you suffer from hypertension,

consult your doctor; a and b remedies are from http://giatroso-
fia -bartzokas.blogspot.gr/.

Hyper-hypothyroidism

In hyperthyroidism (tachycardia, weight loss, anxiety, irritability
and tremor) I use the remote points:

Gb 31, the sharp end of the needle should be pointing towards
the abdomen, dispersion and

Kd 3, the sharp end of the needle should be pointing towards
the big toe, dispersion.

I use a single remote point every day. I also use two local painful
points (right and left) at the anatomical location of thyroid gland
(just below the Adam's apple in the neck).

In hypothyroidism (bradycardia, obesity, apathy) I apply the
general cycle for the stimulation of the kidneys, p. 160.

In case of elevated antithyroid antibodies, I do the same as in
allergy prevention, p. 181 and I also use two local painful points
(right and left) at the anatomical location of thyroid gland (just
below the Adam's apple in the neck).

The above mentioned acupoints are valid when the patient
doesn't take medication or when conventional medical treatment
fails to control the disease.

If the patient is on medication and the disease is well controlled,
then don't insert needles.

Certainly the patient should regularly undergo physical examination, laboratory tests and imaging evaluation.

Remember acupoints for relaxation, p. 119.

Important acupuncture points for hyperthyroidism: Gb 31, Kd 3,
for hypothyroidism: Gb 31, Kd 1, Kd 3.

Herbs for hyperthyroidism: melissa officinalis, lycopus europaeus, verbena officinalis, broccoli, crategus oxyacantha, viscum album, prunella vulgaris, raphanus sativus.

Herbs for hypothyroidism: allium sativum, taraxacum officinalis, petroselinum sativum, leek, orange, walnuts, raphanus sativus (functions well for both hyper and hypothyroidism), glycyrrhiza glabra, beetroot, genista tinctoria, grapes, rubus idaeus.

Example of herb prescription for hyperthyroidism: infusion of melissa officinalis.
Example of herb prescription for hypothyroidism: 1 garlic clove, 3 times daily.

Grandma's remedies:

a. in hypothyroidism apply poultice of hot (tolerable) boiled brassica olarecea on the anatomical location of thyroid gland (just below the Adam's apple in the neck), 3 times daily.

b. in goiter, boil 20g orange tree leaves and blossoms in 1 L water, drink 1 teacup, 2 times daily.

Cupping therapy

Treatment with cups has been applied since ancient times. Horn, pottery, bronze and bamboo cups were used. The origin of cupping therapy is lost back in time and reaches mythological years. Telesphoros, a secondary healing divinity is depicted with a suction cup.

The traditional Hellenic medicine involves the use of cupping. We impregnate a cotton ball with white spirit or alcohol and we firmly fix it on the dents of a fork. We lit it and the flaming cotton ball is then, in one fluid motion, placed into a cup (made from thick glass), quickly removed, and the cup is placed on the skin. As the heated air inside the cup cools, it contracts and draws the skin slightly inside. The cup is left for as long as the period required to heat another cup and to place it symmetrically to the spine in the back.

The treatment is done by placing alternately the two cups (glasses) all over the thorax region of the back (if there are hairs, shave them). Then the patient is covered thoroughly with blanket for at least one hour because the skin pores are open and cold draught can easily penetrate the patient's body. Before starting the cupping therapy, apply olive oil on the skin so that the cups glide easily.

A similar type of cupping called wet or bloody is applied by experts. They do a superficial cut in the sucked skin and they repeat cupping at the same point so as blood to come out (up to 20ml).

There are special cups made from plastic or silicone with a wide range of openings. Vacuum can also be created with a mechanical suction pump acting through a valve located at the top of the cup.

Many Chinese healers place special cups over needles. First they insert a needle, then place a special cup over the needle.

The local heat warms the patient and eliminates the inner cold and dampness.

Cupping is claimed to treat a broad range of medical conditions such as common cold, pneumonia, bronchitis, asthma, pain of rheumatic origin, neuralgia, infertility. Wet cupping is applied to severe pneumonia, poisoning (e.g. locally in case of snake poisoning or in the back in case of poisoning by gases) and hypertensive crisis.

Index of acupoints

Point	Image	Page
Bl 2	6	131
Bl 10	24	185
Bl 40	14	161
Bl 57	14	140
Bl 67	13, 18, 19	138
CV 17	6	121
Du 16	24	185
Extra 1	6	119
Gb 1	6	136
Gb 21	23, 24	171
Gb 31	21, 22	160
Gb 37	22	164
Gb 41	13, 22	228
Gb 44	13, 18, 19	138
HE 1	26	213
Kd 1	20	138
Kd 3	15	161
Kd 10	14	143
LI 1	12	138
LI 4	10	213
LI 15	23	176
LI 20	6	126
Liv 1	13, 17, 19	138

Liv 3	13	235
LU 5	9	126
LU 11	11, 12	138
Pc 6	9	120
Pc 9	11	138
SI1	11, 12	138
SI19	27	134
SJ 1	12	138
SJ 5	10	188
SJ 15	23, 24	171
SJ 17	27	134
SJ 23	6	119
SP 1	15, 17	124
SP 4	15, 16	124
St 9	7	125
St 18	8	243
St 25	8	227
St 31	8	213
St 35	22	167
St 36	13 stimulation, 22 dispersion	123
St 45	13, 17, 19	139

The accompanying video with detailed demonstration of the self acupuncture technique (using one or two hands) and acupuncture points can be watched at **http://youtu.be/358XNqIVPoc**

About the author

Dimitrios P. Mangioros graduated from the Medical Military School and Medical School of the Aristotelian University of Thessaloniki in 1991. He specialized in neurosurgery at the Athens General Hospital "G. Gennimatas". He had a post-graduate education in Germany, at the University Hospital of Cologne, Department of Functional Neurosurgery where he studied peripheral nerve stimulation, deep brain stimulation (for Parkinson's disease, motor disorders, obsessive-compulsive disorder and pain) and stereotactic radiosurgery for brain tumors.

Today, he is a neurosurgeon consultant at the 251 Air Force General Hospital. In addition to his duties as a brain and spine surgeon, he is also in charge of the chronic pain outpatient clinic, where acupuncture, pain relief injections, implantation of electrodes are performed, medications are prescribed and advice on thermal baths and herbs is given.

He has also been trained in nutritional therapy (fasting therapy, fruit therapy, raw food therapy), hypnosis and Shiatsu (massage at acupuncture points).

His favorite sports are winter skiing, windsurfing and trekking. He is married with three children.

Contact details

Private practice: 103 El. Venizelou Avenue, Ilioupoli, 16343, Athens, Greece, Tel: +30 698-351-1330, +30 210-9939665,

e-mail: acumag@hotmail.com

www.ingramcontent.com/pod-product-compliance
Lightning Source LLC
Chambersburg PA
CBHW080551270326
41929CB00019B/3265